The Caregiver's Guide to Cancer

The Caregiver's Guide to Cancer

Compassionate Advice
for Caring for You and
Your Loved One

VICTORIA LANDES, LCSW

ROCKRIDGE
PRESS

For general information on our other products and services or to obtain technical support, please contact our Customer Care Department within the United States at (866) 744-2665, or outside the United States at (510) 253-0500.

Rockridge Press publishes its books in a variety of electronic and print formats. Some content that appears in print may not be available in electronic books, and vice versa.

TRADEMARKS: Rockridge Press and the Rockridge Press logo are trademarks or registered trademarks of Callisto Media Inc. and/or its affiliates, in the United States and other countries, and may not be used without written permission. All other trademarks are the property of their respective owners. Rockridge Press is not associated with any product or vendor mentioned in this book.

Interior and Cover Designer: Lisa Forde
Art Producer: Sue Bischofberger
Editor: Jesse Aylen
Production Editor: Rachel Taenzler
Production Manager: Martin Worthington

Author photo courtesy of Kathy Schwartz

ISBN: Print 978-1-64876-419-6
eBook 978-1-64876-420-2
R0

For the caregivers of the world and the loved ones they cherish.

CONTENTS

Introduction

If you have taken the time to open this book, you are likely one of millions of people worldwide affected by cancer. Perhaps you are the primary caregiver of a cancer survivor or a member of an extended caregiving support network. Whatever way cancer may touch your life, know that you are not alone. Although each caregiver travels their own unique path, there are commonalities that lie at the foundation of the caregiving experience.

A cancer diagnosis can be one of the greatest challenges that humans face. As a caregiver, you may feel hopeless and helpless, striving to find ways to provide sufficient and meaningful support. Caregivers must adapt to the variety of changes that accompany a diagnosis. Providing care can bring fulfillment and closeness, but also emotional, psychological, and physical exhaustion.

A caregiver's commitment to self-care is vital to their health and well-being and will help them provide the best possible support to their loved one. Learning to care for oneself while caring for others can be difficult. Time and energy constraints, feelings of guilt, and lack of resources can all be obstacles to self-care. For these and many other reasons, a desire to be selfless and constantly put the needs of others before one's own is a common thread shared by many caregivers.

I have worked as a licensed clinical social worker in the oncology field for the better part of two decades and have accompanied thousands of patients and caregivers through diagnosis, treatment, caregiving, and survivorship. I have learned that caregiving is a complex experience, and many factors affect a caregiver's ability to balance the demands of the role. To effectively accompany patients and caregivers, it is vital to meet them where they are and work together at a pace that reduces rather than accelerates stress.

This book is intended to serve as an expansive resource for caregivers as they learn to care both for their loved ones and for themselves. Gaining awareness of the various ways a diagnosis can impact one's entire life is an important stepping-stone. Sometimes, it may feel like everything is moving so fast that it is difficult to know what we might need. This book also serves as a guide to understanding and navigating the health-care system, treatments, and side effects; communicating effectively and efficiently with your loved ones and their care team; and managing difficult emotions. It is broken into three parts, each addressing vital aspects of the caregiving journey. Practical advice on what to say, what to do, and what to ask is highlighted in the sidebars included throughout. Caregivers' stories are also showcased, reflecting the knowledge and wisdom they gained along the way. Certain sections may be more relevant to you than others, depending on the unique needs of your particular caregiving scenario, but taken as a whole, this guide is dedicated to you, the caregiver.

Through the years, I've heard caregivers express the value of being seen and heard by others and knowing they are not alone in this experience. May this guide allow you to join millions of caregivers in the collective desire to lovingly support yourself and your loved one through this transformational time.

PART 1

Understanding Cancer

When someone is first diagnosed with cancer, we focus on meeting with doctors to gain knowledge about cancer in general, as well as the patient's unique case. This is also a time to meet the patient's cancer care team, a group of professionals from a variety of disciplines who can aid in diagnosing and treating the cancer and provide emotional and practical support. Caregivers partner with their loved ones to meet new challenges like making difficult decisions, redefining the division of labor in the household, and maintaining open and honest communication.

CHAPTER 1

Cancer Explained

WHITNEY

Isaac remembers getting the call at work from his wife, Whitney. Isaac could hear the concern in her voice when Whitney said, "I found a lump in my breast when I was in the shower this morning. I'm scared." After a series of tests and a biopsy, Whitney received a breast cancer diagnosis. Isaac recalls, "I didn't know what to expect, and everything was happening so fast. I tried to go to work in between medical appointments, but I could barely concentrate. Initially, I was in shock. Whitney was only 38, and this was the furthest thing from our minds. I had no idea what to say or think or do. I wondered how we were going to tell our 10-year-old son."

Whitney's surgeon recommended a mastectomy (breast removal). "I remember this hitting me like a tidal wave," Isaac says. "Whitney and I sat together and cried." After surgery, Whitney went through four rounds of chemotherapy. "I tried to go to every appointment, but some days I had meetings I couldn't miss," Isaac remembers. "I also needed to be there for our son. We have a big network of family and friends, so they helped fill in for me, keeping Whitney company at appointments and doing things for us, like organizing a meal train and running errands. It was hard, and there were good days and bad days. The hardest part was seeing Whitney go through so much, but with all the stories I have heard about cancer, I know we were lucky."

Cancer Defined

In a healthy body, normal cells grow, divide, and eventually die. Cancer is a group of diseases that occur when abnormal cells divide in an uncontrolled manner and do not die. Cancer can start in any cell in the body. These abnormal cells can build up in one location, forming a mass called a tumor. Some cancers form tumors, whereas others, such as leukemia, do not. Tumors can be noncancerous (*benign*) or cancerous (*malignant*). Benign tumors do not invade other areas of the body. Malignant tumors begin growing in one part of the body and can spread to other areas through the blood and lymph systems. Cancer that has spread outside the primary site of growth is called *metastatic cancer*.

Cancer can afflict any person at any point in their life. Although great strides have been made in the treatment of cancer, there are aspects of the disease that have yet to be discovered or understood by scientists. In spite of this, many types of cancer can be successfully treated. In very difficult cases, treatment may be required on an ongoing basis and may eventually stop working.

Why do some people get cancer while others don't? This is a complex question without an easy or clear answer. According to the National Cancer Institute, there are risk factors that can play a role in making a person more vulnerable to cancer:

- **Genetics/family history** can influence inherited susceptibility to cancer.
- **Exposure to cancer-causing substances (*carcinogens*),** such as asbestos, coal, and formaldehyde, can play a role.
- **Advancing age** is a risk factor for many cancers, but not all. For example, leukemia can afflict children and adolescents.
- **The use of hormones** to manage menopausal symptoms can increase the risk for certain types of cancer.
- **Chronic inflammation,** the cause of which is sometimes unknown, can damage DNA and increase cancer risk.

- **Alcohol** consumption is associated with an increased risk for certain cancers, such as liver, breast, and esophageal cancer.
- **Obesity** can contribute to cancer risk.
- **Immunosuppression** (caused by certain medications or disease) can make the immune system less able to detect cancer cells or combat infections that can increase cancer risk.
- **Radiation** can damage DNA, increasing risk for cancer.
- **Sun exposure** can damage the skin, increasing skin cancer risk.
- **Tobacco** in the form of smoking, secondhand smoke, and chewing tobacco can increase cancer risk.

Cancer can be broken into five different categories: carcinoma, sarcoma, melanoma, lymphoma, and leukemia. Although there are over 200 different specific cancers, the most common include melanoma, colorectal cancer, prostate cancer, lung cancer, and breast cancer. The cancer staging process determines the extent of the patient's cancer through a series of medical tests that gauge the advancement of the cancer and whether it has spread to other parts of the body.

Many cancer survivors ask the question, "Why did I get cancer?" Many wonder if they have done something to contribute to their risk. Although there are some risk factors, such as smoking, that appear to have a direct link to cancer risk down the road, there are many cancer survivors who exhibit few or no risk factors. Cancer does not discriminate. Many myths and misconceptions about cancer risk have been given a voice in an effort to explain why some people get it and what their outcome will be, but sometimes the answer is simply: We do not know. Some such common myths include:

- Getting a biopsy makes cancer spread.
- Sugar causes cancer.
- Antiperspirants and deodorants cause breast cancer.
- If a family member has cancer, I will get it, too.
- Cancer is a death sentence.

According to the National Cancer Institute, there is no data to support these myths. Evidence-based science identifies true risk factors and directs treatment recommendations. Some caregivers spend a great deal of time and energy researching the diagnosis. This can be a double-edged sword. Although gaining knowledge can feel empowering, Internet exposure can also needlessly heighten anxiety. There is so much information to sift through, and much of it may not apply to your loved one's situation. Ask your providers to recommend trustworthy Internet sources, and confirm all information with the medical team.

Navigating the initial stages of a cancer diagnosis can be all-consuming and lead to feelings of helplessness. Focusing on quality of life can reduce stress and help you maintain a sense of control. Lifestyle improvements such as good nutrition, adequate rest, hydration, exercise, and stress management can help caregivers and their loved ones maintain physical and emotional resilience throughout the treatment process.

Is This a Sign of Cancer?

When cancer afflicts someone you love, it can create a flurry of feelings, from vulnerability to loss of control and even fear. Certain signs and symptoms can help identify potential health issues in their early stages. It is important to remember that many cancer signs and symptoms can also be caused by less-concerning conditions. If you or a loved one are experiencing any of the following symptoms, follow up with your primary care physician:

- Excessive, ongoing fatigue not caused by lack of sleep
- Pain anywhere in the body that is persistent and/or worsens over time, has no clear cause, and doesn't respond to treatment
- Vaginal bleeding, such as postmenopausal vaginal bleeding or unusual vaginal bleeding in premenopausal women
- Blood in stool and/or black, tarry stool
- Bladder changes, such as pain with urination, frequent urination, blood in urine, or slow urine flow

- Changes in bowel habits, such as ongoing constipation and/or diarrhea or changes in the look of stool
- Breast changes, such as thickening or lumps, bloody nipple discharge, puckering or dimpling of the breast, or inverted nipple
- Bloating that lasts for more than two weeks
- Lumps in testicles
- Inexplicable, persistent cough or hoarseness that does not resolve and is not caused by a respiratory infection
- Changes in moles/warts, such as asymmetrical or multi-colored moles with irregular edges, moles that bleed, or moles that are large and/or growing in size
- Unexpected weight loss
- Stomach pain or nausea lasting two or more weeks
- Night sweats or fevers that persist
- Difficulty swallowing
- Excessive bruising or multiple bruises in unusual places not caused by bumping into objects
- Indigestion, such as heartburn or nausea, lasting more than two weeks
- Abnormal lab work, such as low or high blood counts
- Lumps or swollen lymph nodes that persist
- Chronic headache that persists and/or worsens with time and doesn't respond to medication
- Oral changes such as mouth sores or lesions

Although these symptoms are cause for concern, there are many instances where they are NOT a sign of cancer. A bad headache with no other symptoms is not necessarily a sign of a brain tumor, and fleeting back pain is not likely a sign of bone cancer.

Here are a few things to consider when assessing symptoms:

1. Is the symptom new or intermittent? Usually cancer is more likely if symptoms persist over a period of time.

2. Does the symptom easily resolve with medication? Cancer symptoms tend to be persistent and don't respond well to medication.

3. If you are young (under 40), cancer is less likely to afflict you. However, younger people may be vulnerable to certain cancers, such as blood cancer, lymphomas, colorectal cancer, and testicular cancer. Regardless of age, it is important to see a primary care physician if you are experiencing any of the previously mentioned symptoms.

4. Breast pain is not typically a sign of breast cancer, although if pain persists, following up with your doctor is recommended. Any lump should be evaluated, as should any nipple discharge or a change in the look or feel of the breast or nipple.

5. Constipation without diarrhea or blood in the stool can be a medication-related side effect or a sign that you need to drink more water, change your diet, or engage in more physical movement and exercise. If you have less than three bowel movements per week, you strain to pass stools, or your stools are lumpy or hard, you may be constipated. Contact your doctor if symptoms persist.

What to Ask Your Doctor

1. Discuss your risk factors for cancer (such as family history, smoking, and/or obesity).

2. Ask if any screening tests are recommended, and make sure you are up to date on mammograms, pap smears, and blood work such as Prostate-Specific Antigen (PSA) and Complete Blood Count (CBC) tests.

3. Explain any symptoms you are experiencing, and determine if a workup—such as exams, tests/scans, or blood work—is needed.

4. Discuss any concerns you may have about the effects of stress on your emotional, mental, and physical health. Get input on how to better manage stress.

Diagnosis and Next Steps

How cancer is diagnosed varies greatly and depends on many factors, including the type of cancer as well as the unique presentation of each patient.

The steps leading to a diagnostic workup for cancer can include:

- Presenting to your medical professional with symptoms
- A physical exam by a medical professional that reveals a concerning symptom, such as a breast lump
- Screening tests such as lab tests, mammograms, CT and/or MRI scans, colonoscopies, and pap smears

If tests come back abnormal and are concerning, a biopsy is done to rule out cancer. There are many different types of biopsies, including needle, endoscopic, and surgical. The tissue sample taken during the biopsy is sent to a pathologist, a medical doctor with expertise in identifying abnormalities in tissue samples and bodily fluids. The pathologist writes a pathology report, which describes the findings in detail and is a critical part of making a cancer diagnosis. Pathologists are an integral part of any cancer care team.

When someone you love deeply is given a cancer diagnosis, the cascade of thoughts and emotions varies from person to person. Some people feel flooded with worry, fear, and sadness, while others may feel shock, disbelief, detachment, or numbness. Sometimes the person receiving the diagnosis may react in one way while their loved ones have their own differing responses. All reactions are valid in this delicate situation.

The time surrounding the initial diagnosis can be particularly overwhelming and anxiety-inducing, especially because it may take time to get a complete diagnosis and treatment recommendations. For example, a breast cancer survivor often does not know if they will need chemotherapy until after surgery is done and the pathology report is completed. That process can take several weeks or longer. Managing the stress of this particularly difficult period can be challenging for all involved. Concerns can arise about missing work, managing the household, and losing income. It can be a sobering time of getting in touch with life's precarious nature and one's own mortality. Some may experience deep feelings of grief and sadness, anticipating the changes and losses that may be approaching.

No matter the stage, for many a cancer diagnosis is a crisis that calls for a mobilization of resources on all levels. Managing the deluge of emotions coupled with the practical demands of planning for treatment can be exhausting. Caregivers can feel an overwhelming sense of responsibility and face uncertainty about how to prioritize the needs of the patient and family. In these initial stages, taking control and getting thoughtfully organized can help diminish those feelings of helplessness.

Some of the tasks may include:

- Making and attending appointments for further testing (if applicable) and meeting your cancer care team
- Obtaining a second opinion, if desired
- Adjusting work and home schedules
- Applying for disability and family leave (FMLA)
- Arranging for child, pet, and family care as needed
- Researching the diagnosis and available treatment options using trustworthy sources, such as the National Comprehensive Cancer Network website (NCCN.org under "Patient Resources"), to better under-stand and anticipate your loved one's needs
- Mobilizing your support network and delegating tasks
- Communicating with your support network about the diagnosis and recommended treatment
- Seeking out cancer support professionals who can pro-vide information, counseling, and care coordination and help you navigate the health-care system

Sometimes there is so much to accomplish in day-to-day life that caregivers are forced to put their emotions on hold. Be excep-tionally kind to yourself. Remember that there is only so much one can accomplish in a day, and let that be enough. Whoever wishes to help in some way, let them. The saying "It takes a village" could not be more relevant than it is in cancer care. Caring for someone going through cancer is more of a marathon than a sprint. Accepting help will create space to better tend to your loved one, your relationship, and yourself.

How Are You Doing?

As a caregiver, it can be difficult to integrate self-care into your life. Before the diagnosis, you may have had a variety of stress-reducing mechanisms like exercise, hobbies, dining out, and spending time with family and friends. Although these outlets may no longer be accessible due to time constraints and the stresses of treatment and appointments, there are other ways to help manage stress that can make a difference. Consider doing a daily 5- to 10-minute relaxation practice like a breathing exercise. Under stress, breathing can become shallow and rapid, and it may be difficult to get a deep, cleansing breath.

- Sit or lie down in a quiet place, if you can find one.
- Breathe in and out slowly through your nose.
- Count each inhalation and exhalation, making sure your breathing is even.
- Focus on your breathing and counting.
- For deeper breathing, inhale through your nose and hold for five counts, then slowly exhale.

If sitting quietly is difficult, consider mindful movement activities, like stretching, gentle yoga, or a short walk. The amount of time you spend on the activity is less important than the act of relaxation itself. Though you may not be the one with the diagnosis, you also deserve care, self-compassion, and understanding. Now, let's explore the journey of caregiving together.

CHAPTER 2

A Caregiver's Journey Begins

SEBASTIAN

Sebastian and Maria had just celebrated their 50th wedding anniversary when Sebastian was diagnosed with multiple myeloma. He had been experiencing some pain near his ribs for a couple of months, but it was manageable and not terribly concerning. In the days following their anniversary, Sebastian began to experience considerably more pain that was not responding to over-the-counter medication. His doctor ordered a workup. A few days later, Sebastian's doctor called to tell him he had multiple myeloma.

Over their years of marriage, Maria and Sebastian had worked extremely well as a team. Their relationship was one of interdependence, with each doing their part to manage daily life. Maria recalls, "After Sebastian was diagnosed, every role shifted and changed. I had to take over everything, and decisions that we had once made together became my sole responsibility. I wanted to do the right thing and everything possible to make him better." Maria remembers how steep the learning curve was and how each day presented new challenges. She had to come to terms not only with her new roles and responsibilities but also with the loss of the man she once knew. "At times during treatment, Sebastian wasn't up to participating in making decisions or taking part in our day-to-day life," Maria remembers. "But throughout this process, I did what I had to do. I didn't know I had the strength to carry it all, but somehow I found it."

Changing Relationships

A cancer diagnosis can bring about a whirlwind of change. Roles and responsibilities, emotional and physical intimacy, and communication needs can all shift dramatically for both patient and caregiver. Although adapting to such change often brings challenges, it can also provide opportunities for growth and greater fulfillment.

The demands of treatment often mean a shift in work hours and schedules and may result in a significant loss of income. Caregivers may need to work more hours or find alternate income sources to bridge the gap. Responsibilities within the family, such as domestic duties, managing finances, and child-rearing, may also need to shift. Sometimes, when a child is the caregiver for a parent, there is an inherent role reversal that can feel unnatural and challenge the relationship unexpectedly. In some family systems, cultural beliefs drive roles and responsibilities. For example, in some cultures, females are relied upon as family caregivers. Some cultures look to men to provide for the family. These dynamics may change after a cancer diagnosis and create an imbalance in the family structure.

At times, the person going through treatment may be too tired or overwhelmed to participate fully in their care, and the caregiver may have to communicate with medical professionals and make important health-care decisions. This dynamic may work well for some, but it can be stressful for others.

Feelings of loss of control, fear, sadness, anger, and frustration are all common and can strain relationships. As a caregiver, you may even feel guilty, as these feelings may not seem justified when juxtaposed with your loved one's suffering. These feelings are very common among caregivers. Finding outlets for self-care is critical for your health and balance, as well as your ability to stay strong for your loved ones. Feeling self-centered for taking care of yourself is understandable, as we all want to try to do everything possible to make our loved ones well. However, without taking proper care of yourself, you will eventually find yourself overwhelmed and depleted, perhaps putting your own health and well-being in jeopardy.

The stress and strain of treatment can also make it difficult to communicate, so extra effort may be needed to speak sensitively and openly. Some people may find it difficult to contain their emotions, while others may withdraw. The perspectives you each hold and the lens through which you view life may be quite different, but all perspectives are equally valid and should be respected. Finding outlets to express your emotions and needs is of the utmost importance. Many find support and comfort talking to friends, family members, spiritual advisors, or mental health professionals.

Physical and emotional intimacy may also diminish due to factors like side effects from treatments or emotional fallout from the stress. Sometimes the side effects are such that caregivers feel they have "lost" their loved one. Treatment can affect sexual health as well, triggering depression, fatigue, and a variety of other symptoms that may make intimacy more difficult.

Relationships with friends and other family members may also change. Many caregivers are naturally more comfortable in the giving role. Accepting and asking for help may feel uncomfortable. It is important to face this discomfort and receive support, whether in a practical form, such as meals, errands, or transportation, or emotional support through time with family and friends, professional counseling, or a support group.

While navigating a cancer diagnosis can be extremely stressful, it can also provide opportunities to deepen relationships and establish more intimate connections. Some describe this time as creating a closeness they hadn't previously experienced. When adversity is faced with good support and open communication, shared bonds can grow stronger. Although future plans may have to be put on hold and visions and dreams may go unfulfilled, priorities may shift, allowing for a time of learning to be present, fully savoring every moment, and cherishing your experiences together.

What to Do

- Communicate as openly and sensitively as possible. Good communication lies at the foundation of close, healthy relationships.

- Understand that people have different ways of coping with challenges. Make an effort to respect the coping styles of others, and be sure to honor your own.

- Try to make self-care a priority. Good nutrition, exercise, rest, quiet time, and social contact are vital to your mental and physical health.

- Engage in prayer/meditation/spiritual practices if you find them helpful.

- Find people to talk to about your feelings and experiences as a caregiver. Accept offers of help and support.

- Join a caregiver support group.

- Consider asking a trusted person to communicate information to your support network. Check the Resources section (see page 158) for more information.

- Seek out social workers, cancer care coordinators, and other mental health professionals who provide services such as counseling and who can connect your family with invaluable community resources.

Long-Distance Caregiving

Caregiving from a distance adds a unique set of challenges to an already trying situation. All the tasks that need to be accomplished must either be done remotely or through local resources. Mobilizing care can require significantly more time and energy in the way of research and phone calls, and finances may be taxed by missed work and travel expenses.

When caregivers cannot attend medical appointments in person, they must manage medical care via phone or email. Obtaining permission to discuss your loved one's medical situation with their providers is of paramount importance. This is done through a Release of Information Form signed by the patient. The oncology practice can assist with executing this form. There also may come a time when your loved one may not be able to make their own health-care decisions. Having a health-care directive, also known as a Durable Power of Attorney for Health Care, in place allows patients to appoint a trusted person (known as a health-care surrogate) to step in and make decisions if needed. Many designate their spouse or partner, another family member, or a close friend. This form can be found online or through your health-care provider. Typically, either a notary or two witnesses are required at the time of signature, but a lawyer does not need to be present.

If you are responsible for managing finances, accessing bank accounts, and paying bills, it will be helpful for your loved one to execute a Durable Power of Attorney for Finances, which can also be found online. See the Resources section (page 158) for organizations that can provide more information on these legal forms.

If the resources are available, create a local support network. Mobilize any family members, friends, and community allies who can assist with caregiving tasks. Pick a trusted person to be your eyes and ears to check in on your loved one. Give them access to the home in case of an emergency. Stay organized and keep local helpers updated so they can provide appropriate support.

Some long-distance caregivers may not be available on a daily basis for all necessary care coordination efforts. Hiring a local care manager can take the load off considerably. Care managers are professionals, such as nurses or social workers, who can serve as advocates or mediators and assist with difficult decisions, such as determining when a higher level of care may be necessary. They can also help with hiring in-home caregivers and executing important legal and financial documents.

Another valuable resource for safety and peace of mind is a medical alert system, also known as a remote monitoring system.

With your loved one's permission, consider installing one in case of an emergency. Many companies provide these services, which can be easily accessed at the push of a button and will send help.

Long-distance caregivers may experience deeper levels of grief, having to rely on hired help and not being able to connect with their loved one as often in person. Try to spend as much quality time together as possible. If you have access to video technology, use it. Being able to see your loved one in real time can enhance feelings of comfort and closeness. If you have a disagreement, attempt to work it out or let it go. Offer your listening ear, as listening empathetically is one of the greatest gifts you can offer.

What to Do

- Establish a good connection with the medical team. Determine the best people to speak with in the oncology practice, such as medical assistants, nurse practitioners, or cancer care coordinators.

- Execute a Durable Power of Attorney for Health Care and a Durable Power of Attorney for Finances.

- Create a local support network of family, friends, and allies.

- Consider hiring a local care management agency.

- Consider installing a remote monitoring system.

- Determine your employer's paid time off (PTO) and Family Medical Leave Act (FMLA) policies so you can plan your visits.

- When you visit, have a list of goals to accomplish so you can budget your time accordingly.

- Most important, spend as much quality time as possible with your loved one, both remotely and in person.

Working with a Cancer Care Team

Your loved one has received a cancer diagnosis, and suddenly you find yourself in the throes of trying to navigate a complicated health-care system. Assimilating new information can feel intimidating and overwhelming. It's not just about visiting with doctors and learning about the diagnosis and treatment. A holistic approach to cancer care that addresses your loved one's physical, mental, emotional, and spiritual needs is vital.

A cancer care team consists of a variety of professionals who specialize in diagnosing, treating, and supporting cancer patients and their loved ones. Many health institutions establish cancer centers that are able to provide comprehensive care under one roof, giving patients easier access to services. All cancer care programs must meet certain standards, and many are accredited by the American College of Surgeons' Commission on Cancer.

The cancer care team encourages the involvement of caregivers in all aspects of care. From attending medical appointments to meeting with the cancer care coordinator or joining your loved one in a support group, caregivers are essential members of the team. Understanding the role of each team member is critical to getting optimal care. Because your loved one may be very busy undergoing care and managing side effects, it may be up to you to seek out help from the care team. Your role may be that of information gatherer, researcher, advocate, and care coordinator. It's important to remember that you are not alone in wanting the best for your loved one. Your cancer care team is there to assist and guide you in this process.

Good communication lies at the heart of the cancer caregiving experience. Learn early on how best to access and communicate with your team members to get the information you need.

These care professionals may be a part of your team:

Medical Oncologist

A medical oncologist is a medical doctor who specializes in the diagnosis and treatment of cancer. They are experts in various treatments, including chemotherapy, biological therapy, hormone therapy, and targeted therapy. The medical oncologist is central to the care process, overseeing treatment and coordination with the team.

Radiologist

A radiologist is a medical doctor who utilizes a variety of imaging procedures to help diagnose and treat cancer. These procedures include X-ray, CT, MRI, PET, and ultrasound scans. Interventional radiologists use image-guided techniques to deliver targeted treatment plans. Radiologists can also subspecialize in certain areas, such as breast imaging.

Surgeon

General surgeons and surgical oncologists diagnose and treat cancer through a variety of surgical procedures. Cancer is treated by removing tumors and nearby tissues that may be cancerous. The difference between a general surgeon and a surgical oncologist is the length and type of training the person has undergone. Your cancer team can help determine if a surgical oncologist is needed.

Radiation Oncologist

Radiation oncologists have specialized training in treating many different types of cancer with radiation using external and/or internal radiation sources to kill cancer cells. Radiation oncologists are also experts in mitigating and managing the side effects of radiation.

Pathologist

Pathologists are medical doctors who use laboratory methods to detect and diagnose diseases. When a biopsy or surgery is performed, pathologists analyze the tissues and fluids and com-municate their findings in a pathology report. Pathology reports are key to determining the extent of disease present, as well as the most effective treatment methods.

Oncology Nurse

Oncology nurses are registered nurses who provide comprehensive cancer care, including assessment, education, care coordination, and administration of treatments. They play a vital role in assessing and managing treatment side effects and provide emotional support and comfort to patients and their loved ones.

Cancer Care Coordinator

Those in a cancer care coordinator support role, like health navigators and social workers, have a diverse set of responsibilities. Ideally, their involvement begins at the time of initial diagnosis, and they follow a patient's care through treatment and into survivorship. They provide information and clarification regarding diagnoses and treatments; facilitate communication; provide care coordination, advocacy, and counseling services; and run support groups.

Nutritionist/Registered Dietician

Nutritionists guide patients and families regarding diet, finding optimal ways to support the body during and after treatment. They can provide guidance on mitigating side effects during treatment, particularly those related to digestion.

Physical Therapist

Physical therapists provide support through a variety of movement approaches, both during and after cancer treatment. Movement is a key part of supporting overall health, mitigating treatment side effects, and boosting the immune system. Some physical therapists specialize in the treatment of lymphedema, which is a possible side effect of some cancer treatments such as surgery and radiation.

What to Do

- Upon diagnosis, seek out the cancer care coordinator. This team member can fill you in on the entire cancer care process and introduce the roles of the other team members.

- Identify the best point of contact for each provider, such as medical assistants and nurse practitioners who can help facilitate communication.

- Learn the communication protocols for each provider. Obtain important contact information like phone numbers, office locations, and email addresses.

- Tell the team members what you are trying to accomplish and ask for their support.

- Consider a friendly rather than confrontational approach when communicating with the care team.

- Appoint one person in your support network to communicate with medical professionals.

- When speaking with doctors, have your list of questions ready and try to ask all the questions at one time rather than in a rolling fashion.

- Be proactive in seeking out needed services. Although care team members are there to help, they cannot always anticipate every patient's needs.

What to Ask Your Care Team

1. What is the diagnosis, i.e., the type and staging?

2. What are the treatment recommendations?

3. What is the expected timeline for treatment?

4. What are the goals of treatment?

5. How soon should treatment start?

6. What are the short- and long-term side effects of the treatment, and how are they best managed?

7. What other medical providers will be involved in the care?

8. Is genetic counseling recommended?

9. What advice do you have for navigating information on the Internet? Are there sites and information sources you recommend?

10. How are second opinions obtained?

11. Can you explain clinical trials? Are they applicable?

12. What support services are available?

13. What is the best way to communicate with you, both directly and with your office?

How Are You Doing?

Although it may be difficult as a caregiver to think about your own needs, even short periods of downtime can make a significant difference in your ability to cope with the stresses of caregiving. Try to budget time for activities such as exercise, connecting with supportive family and friends, and your own health-related appointments.

When you're feeling stressed, take a few minutes to try this mindfulness exercise:

- Sit down in a quiet place and take a few deep breaths.
- As your breathing slows, think about a time in your life when you felt relaxed and content.
- Allow the images of the scene to become more vivid. Recall the colors, sounds, and smells.
- Allow the feelings of contentment and relaxation to come over you as you see yourself in this peaceful place.
- Repeat this exercise anytime you want to invoke feelings of peace and relaxation.

PART 2

Caring for Someone with Cancer

Following a diagnosis, attention quickly turns to the patient. Caregivers often wonder how they can best support their loved one and need a road map to help them navigate these uncharted waters. Although every case requires a uniquely tailored treatment plan, getting educated about common side effects and management strategies can be helpful. It is also prudent to prepare for common shifts in daily schedules and household logistics, nutrition and lifestyle habits, roles and responsibilities, and communication and intimacy.

CHAPTER 3

Treatments and Side Effects

MIKE

Jasmine's husband, Mike, was diagnosed with stage III colon cancer at the age of 45. Jasmine was in shock when she found out the cancer had spread to Mike's lymph nodes and he would need 12 rounds of chemotherapy and radiation. "In the beginning, everything was too fast and too extreme," Jasmine says. "You have to complete that first treatment, then it becomes normal and a lot of the fear dissipates."

Some day-to-day roles remained the same, but Jasmine took over all the shopping, cooking, and cleaning. "I enjoyed this, as I love to cook and meal plan." She also spent a good deal of time researching how to manage the side effects Mike was experiencing. "Sometimes we clashed over what to do," she explains. "I didn't realize that Mike needed to do certain things to manage his anxiety. When I finally understood better what he was going through, it helped me let go and stop pushing. Mike made a huge effort to stay busy and active, and I realized this was what helped him the most." For Mike, some of the more challenging side effects were constipation, insomnia, and all-consuming emotions like anger, frustration, and fear. Jasmine recalls how Mike took a "holistic approach and got involved with Buddhism, a support group, and even met a fellow cancer survivor who became his life coach. You realize that help comes in many different forms."

Common Cancer Treatments

The world of cancer treatment is vast, complex, and ever-changing. Your loved one will have an individualized treatment plan, one tailored to their specific scenario, which may include one or more of the following:

Surgery

Surgery is used as a primary treatment for many types of cancer. It involves removing the cancerous tumor and nearby tissues through an operation performed by a general surgeon or surgical oncologist. It is important that nearby tissues (including a small amount of healthy tissue) be removed in order to ensure all the cancer is gone. Surgery may also involve removing nearby lymph nodes to determine whether the cancer has spread.

Radiation Therapy

Radiation therapy uses a high level of radiation to eradicate cancer cells. Sometimes it's the only treatment needed, although it can also be used in conjunction with surgery, chemotherapy, and immunotherapy. There are different types of radiation, including external beam radiation, brachytherapy, and systemic radiation therapy. Sometimes radiation therapy is used to relieve symptoms in a palliative care setting. There is a limit to how much radiation the body can receive in a lifetime, and that limit may vary from person to person.

Chemotherapy

Chemotherapy uses drugs to kill cancer cells. Some chemotherapy drugs are taken orally in the form of pills or liquids, whereas others are infused into the body using an intravenous (IV) catheter. Chemotherapy can also be given by injection into the muscle or directly into a body cavity, or it can be applied topically with cream or ointment. Chemotherapy targets all fast-growing cells, such as those that form tumors. Chemotherapy drugs can be given as single agents or as a combination of drugs. Each chemotherapy drug carries potential side effects, ranging from fatigue and digestive disturbance to mood, appetite, and cognitive changes.

Immunotherapy

Immunotherapy helps the body better fight cancer. When the immune system is functioning well, it can help prevent or slow cancer growth. Under the umbrella of biological therapy, there are several different types of immunotherapy. It is given in various forms, such as oral, topical, intravenous, and intravesical (directly into the bladder). Although several immunotherapy drugs have been approved to treat certain types of cancer, chemotherapy, surgery, and radiation remain the more widely used treatments.

Targeted Therapy

This type of cancer treatment identifies "targets" within cells and interferes with the growth of cancer. Although chemotherapy seeks to kill cells, targeted therapy acts on specific characteristics of cells associated with cancer growth, thereby halting or slowing the disease's progression. There are many different types of targeted therapies, and their applicability depends on whether or not a person's tumor has a specific, eligible target.

Hormone Therapy

Hormonally driven cancers, like breast and prostate cancer, can be treated with hormone therapy. Also known as "endocrine therapy," hormone therapy typically reduces the overall amount of a hormone in the body or blocks the action the hormone has on cancer cells. Hormone therapy is typically used alongside other treatments and can help reduce the risk of cancer recurrence.

Stem Cell Transplant

Also known as bone marrow transplants, stem cell transplants treat certain types of cancer that affect bone marrow, like leukemia, lymphoma, and myeloma. Cancer and cancer treatment can damage bone marrow, which can affect critical functions like the production of white blood cells, red blood cells, and platelets. A stem cell transplant takes healthy cells and transplants them into the bone marrow, helping restore immune function.

Medication

Medications can be used for cancer treatment and to help mitigate side effects such as allergic reactions, nausea and vomiting, constipation and diarrhea, pain, neutropenia (low white blood cell count), mouth sores, sleep problems, anxiety, depression, and low appetite.

What to Ask Your Doctor

1. What is the total length of time anticipated for treatment?

2. How many rounds of treatment are planned?

3. How many days/weeks are between each round of treatment?

4. Will the treatment be given orally, through IV, or through another method, such as injection?

5. What are some of the anticipated side effects, and what are resources for managing them (for example, infusion center nurses who may be available for telephone advice)?

6. What symptoms should be reported immediately?

7. What is the success rate of the recommended treatment?

8. What Internet sources do you recommend for learning about the treatment regimen and managing side effects?

Common Side Effects

Although every patient has a unique experience, some side effects are common. Be sure to call your oncologist or the infusion center staff about any side effects that you're having difficulty managing. Keep important information sheets from the doctor and infusion center, especially on symptoms requiring immediate attention, such as fever, shortness of breath, or changes in mental status.

Anxiety and Depression

From the moment of diagnosis, feelings like shock, fear, sadness, frustration, and anger can arise. Fear of the unknown and the overwhelming responsibility of navigating treatment can produce anxiety. Many survivors experience life changes and losses that can also lead to depression. Treatment is physically taxing, and some medications may exacerbate anxiety and depression.

What to Say

"Naturally you feel overwhelmed and anxious right now. This is a very challenging time, but we are in this together, and I'm here to support you."

"I know there is a lot for you to contend with right now. If you feel overwhelmed and scared sometimes, that's really understandable. You are handling this so well."

"Your body is going through so much, and many things in your life have had to change because of this. If you'd like to talk, I'm here to listen."

"I imagine this is common during treatment. Maybe the doctor can offer some suggestions."

What to Do

- Provide opportunities to talk, actively listen with empathy, and validate your loved one's feelings. Sometimes people need to vent and be heard and aren't looking for advice.

- Encourage getting out and doing something enjoyable.

- Suggest movement, such as walking or stretching.

- If your loved one is connected to spiritual practices such as church/temple attendance, meditation, or prayer, encourage greater participation in those activities.

- Ask if talking to a counselor/therapist might be helpful, and facilitate connection to those resources.

- If you feel your loved one may be open to it, bring up the topic of support groups. Talk about potential benefits, such as hearing how others are coping with treatment and dealing with loneliness and isolation.

- If symptoms are persistent, talk about the possibility of using medication to help. Suggest they discuss their concerns with their oncologist/primary care doctor or request a referral to psychological services for consultation.

What to Ask Your Doctor

1. What advice do you have for managing anxiety and/or depression?

2. How will we know if medication is needed?

3. If medication is warranted, will you prescribe it yourself or provide a referral?

4. Could the treatment medications be causing the anxiety and/or depression? If so, when do you anticipate a shift in symptoms?

5. What about diet? Can you provide a referral to someone who is well versed in nutrition and how it relates to anxiety and/or depression?

Appetite Loss

Treatment side effects can cause appetite loss for a variety of reasons. Some patients can lose their sense of taste or experience an unpleasant taste in the mouth, and some foods may not taste the same as they once did. Dry mouth is also very common and can affect the desire to eat, as can mouth sores. Remedies for these side effects include medications and mouthwashes, as well as shifts in exercise habits, nutrition, and social contact.

What to Say

"I was doing some reading about appetite loss, and there are some things we can do to make this better."

"The doctor may have some ideas on how to help. There are medications they use to increase appetite."

"The treatment is causing [taste changes, a bad taste, mouth sores], and that could be a big part of why you don't feel like eating. Let's talk to the doctor about this."

"Let's talk to a nutritionist about ways to increase appetite and add more calories to your diet."

What to Do

- Ask your loved one if they are having mouth-related side effects such as a loss of taste, bad taste, or mouth sores.

- Encourage small meals every two to three hours. Smaller amounts of food are easier to eat and digest.

- Have easy-to-eat, healthy snacks on hand that are nutrient-dense and higher in calories and protein.

- Contact a nutritionist who specializes in oncology care.

- Consider limiting foods that are greasy, heavy, or produce a lot of gas, such as Brussels sprouts, cabbage, broccoli, and cauliflower.

- Encourage an increase in fluid intake with water and herbal teas. Suggest limiting alcohol, which can irritate mouth sores and be hard on the liver, as well as caffeinated beverages, which can be dehydrating.

- Through trial and error, determine what foods are most palatable.

- Sometimes changing the dining environment can help. Try eating with friends and family and presenting food in a more colorful and pleasing way. Become aware of the smells, sights, and sounds that are most appetite-inducing for your loved one.

What to Ask Your Doctor

1. Is there a prescription mouthwash for mouth sores? What over-the-counter remedies do you recommend?

2. Can you please provide a referral to a nutritionist?

3. Are there any medications to consider to stimulate appetite?

4. Is it okay to exercise to help stimulate appetite? What type of exercise do you recommend?

Cognitive Changes

Some people experience cognitive changes (also known as "chemo brain") that can include difficulty focusing, fogginess, lack of concentration, and inability to remember certain things. It can be very disconcerting not to be able to do things that once came easily. Most cognitive changes are short-term and typically resolve after treatment ends, but some can be long-term depending on the cause, such as when cancer affects the brain.

What to Say

"I can only imagine how hard it must be to not feel like yourself."

"The doctors and nurses said you might experience this and it's very common with treatment."

"I know you are used to multitasking and keeping up with everything. You are doing amazingly well considering how much of your energy is needed to process your treatment."

"How can I help? I am happy to pick up some extra tasks so you can focus on healing."

"Maybe there are some other activities you'd like to do that don't require so much focus, like taking more walks or catching up on that series you said you wanted to watch."

What to Do

- Normalize cognitive changes and remind your loved one that this is a common experience with cancer treatment.

- Actively listen to their concerns. Call the doctor if the cognitive changes are alarming or seem beyond what you were told you should expect.

- Repeat information as often as necessary.

- Point out how well they are doing considering the demands of treatment.

- Help them manage their life in an organized fashion. Encourage note-taking. Post notes as reminders. Use files to keep track of important information.

- Join your loved one in a relaxing meditation or yoga practice or take walks together.

- Facilitate connection with resources like exercise programs and support groups.

- Encourage activities that require more concentration at times when they are feeling their best.

- If your loved one is up to it, encourage them to engage in memory-enhancing activities, such as crossword puzzles, sudoku, and other brain exercises.

What to Ask Your Doctor

1. These cognitive changes are really hard. How can we tell if they are related to treatment and not caused by another problem?

2. Are there other conditions that could be causing these memory problems?

3. Do you need to run other tests or provide a referral to other providers in order to rule out other conditions?

4. Is there anything we can do to make this better or at least stabilize it?

Delirium

Delirium is a mental state characterized by confusion. It can be accompanied by restlessness, reduced awareness of surroundings, and delusions or hallucinations. Cancer patients can experience delirium as a result of the cancer itself or from treatment side effects. Other possible causes of delirium include medication side effects, infections, dehydration, lack of sleep, low or high blood sugar, and pain. There is a higher incidence of delirium in advanced cancer and at the end of life.

What to Say

"I want to encourage you to rest."

"I'm here to help make you more comfortable."

"I want to reassure you that I am here. You are not alone. You are safe."

"Would you like to get up and sit in a chair? It may feel good to change your position."

What to Do

- Call the doctor immediately to report a shift in mental status, such as confusion, paranoia, depression, delusions, or hallucinations.

- Keep the room/house quiet and calm.

- Speak very clearly and with few words. It is easier for your loved one to process simple language.

- Do not argue over what is true or correct, as this can be agitating.

- Keep your loved one comfortable. Offer to help them sit up in a chair, if desired.

- If they feel up to eating or drinking, help facilitate that.

- Explain where they are.

- Read books, letters, or email messages aloud—anything personal to them. This can be calming and help your loved one feel connected.

- Try playing soothing music and see if that is enjoyable.

- If not at home, bring familiar items such as pillows and pictures to make them more comfortable.

What to Ask Your Doctor

1. What is the possible cause(s) of the delirium?

2. What tests, if any, are needed to determine the cause?

3. Is this a result of the cancer itself, some other cause, or both?

4. What can be done to minimize agitation and maximize comfort?

5. Are there any medications that can help?

6. Are there any other services that might be helpful, such as a physical therapist or occupational therapist?

7. Should 24-hour supervision be considered?

Fatigue

Fatigue is one of the most common side effects, characterized by a feeling of exhaustion and/or weakness, and it can be so extreme that it inhibits a person's ability to engage in normal daily life. Although tiredness improves with rest and sleep, fatigue does not improve even after a full night's rest. Fatigue sometimes gets better or worse during treatment, depending on where someone is in the cycle.

What to Say

"What can I do to help lighten your load so you can rest more?"

"I can see this fatigue is really affecting you. Let's talk to the doctor. Sometimes there are other things going on that may cause fatigue, like low iron levels."

"If you'd like, I can help you organize your day so you don't take on too much and have time to take care of yourself. If there's any time to focus on self-care, it's now."

"I have been doing some research, and it looks like there are things you can do to improve your energy during treatment. If and when you want to talk about it, I am here."

What to Do

- Validate and normalize your loved one's feelings by listening and acknowledging their experience.

- If you are concerned about the level of fatigue or you suspect that there may be other contributing issues, call the doctor. Fatigue can be caused by several other conditions, such as anemia, stress, depression, decreased nutrition, poor sleep, reactions to medications, poor hydration, and pain.

- Ask what you can do to help. Offer to take on additional responsibilities.

- Delegate tasks to your support network.

- Get educated on managing fatigue. Encourage your loved one to consult with a dietician on ways to increase their intake of calories and nutrient-dense foods. Encourage optimal fluid intake.

- Encourage movement, such as walking, stretching, or other more rigorous forms of exercise, if tolerated.

- Consider integrative therapies that can help combat fatigue, such as acupuncture and acupressure.

What to Ask Your Doctor

1. Can you tell me what red flags I should be aware of that might point to other possible causes of fatigue?

2. Are there tests to rule out other causes of fatigue?

3. Do you have any dietary recommendations to combat fatigue? Can we have a referral to a dietician?

4. My loved one is experiencing other symptoms (such as increased anxiety, depression, and/or overwhelming stress). Do you recommend a referral to a counselor/therapist and/or psychiatrist for a medication evaluation?

5. We are considering trying out some integrative therapies such as acupuncture. Do you have any recommendations?

Hair Loss

When someone finds out that chemotherapy is recommended for them, they often wonder how they will cope with losing their hair. It changes one's appearance, making the cancer diagnosis visible.

Going through treatment anonymously is no longer possible. Many people greatly value their hair as part of their identity and can feel exposed or experience a great sense of loss. Not all chemotherapy causes hair loss, and some drugs may only cause partial hair loss or thinning. Chemotherapy-related hair loss is typically temporary, and the hair will usually grow back after treatment. Some people use scalp-cooling "cold caps" to preserve their hair. These caps diminish the amount of chemotherapy medications that reach the hair follicles.

What to Say

"There's a lot of great information out there on how to deal with hair loss. You can get a wig or use hats and scarves. I can take you to some shops to look around, if you'd like."

"The American Cancer Society does a workshop called 'Look Good, Feel Better.' It looks like a great place to get tips on dealing with hair loss. I can get more information and sign you up, if you'd like."

"Maybe we can look into the cold caps and see if we can preserve your hair through treatment. We'll need to talk to the doctor about this and see if it's an option."

What to Do

- Let your loved one start the conversation about hair loss. If they are sad about it, acknowledge that hair loss can cause grief. Listen and validate their feelings.

- Do not try to enroll them in feeling upbeat. Experiencing hair loss is very difficult and may feel traumatic for some.

- Before hair begins to fall out, suggest getting a shorter cut. Watching hair fall out in clumps can feel distressing and traumatic.

- Research local wig shops, which also typically sell hats and scarves. Offer to take your loved one shopping.

- Support whatever decisions your loved one makes about coping with their hair loss. Some decide to wear nothing, while others may feel it's important to always wear something.

- Offer compliments frequently.

What to Ask Your Doctor

1. Does the chemotherapy regimen cause hair loss?

2. If so, will all hair fall out or will it just thin?

3. When does hair typically start to fall out?

4. When does it start growing back?

5. What about cold caps? Are they a good idea in this situation? If so, what are the infusion center's capabilities with this technology?

6. Is it okay to dye hair once it has grown back some?

7. What resources do you recommend for coping with hair loss?

Incontinence

Incontinence refers to the involuntary loss of bladder or bowel control. It can be caused by cancer itself or by some cancer treatments. Some cancers and treatments are more likely to cause incontinence. For example, radiation to the pelvic, abdominal, or genital areas can increase risk of incontinence. Approaches to managing incontinence include surgery, medications, incontinence products, pelvic floor strengthening, and training programs.

What to Say

"I'm here to listen if ever you want to share how you are doing with this."

"I think the doctor may have some suggestions as to how to manage this. I can make an appointment if you are up to that, or we can try calling them."

"Whatever we need to do, I will help in any way I can."

What to Do

- Listen empathetically. Let your loved one know you want to be a sounding board if and when they want to talk about it.

- Process your own feelings with friends or family.

- Educate yourself through doctor-recommended literature or reliable websites.

- Help your loved one regain some control by pursuing actions that may remedy the problem.

- Learn which foods and drinks exacerbate their condition.

- Consider waterproofing furniture.

- Obtain incontinence products such as pads, adult diapers, or sheet protectors as needed.

- Consider getting equipment such as a raised toilet seat or bedside commode if appropriate. A room deodorizer may also be helpful.

- Consider contacting a continence specialist.

What to Ask Your Doctor

1. What is causing the incontinence?

2. What are your recommendations for managing it?

3. Is there a procedure or medication that can help?

4. What about a bladder/bowel training program?

5. Would a referral to a physical therapist be helpful for pelvic floor strengthening?

6. What kind of supplies should we get and where?

7. Is this expected to get better with time?

8. How will we know when we need to bring equipment into the house, such as a raised toilet seat or a bedside commode?

Constipation/Diarrhea

Constipation and diarrhea refer to an imbalance in the digestive system that can lead to a variety of symptoms. Constipation is characterized by infrequent or incomplete bowel movements, hard stools, or difficulty passing stools. Diarrhea is characterized by loose, watery bowel movements occurring three or more times in a day. In cancer care, constipation and diarrhea are common problems with a variety of potential causes. Each has its own set of remedies, including medications and dietary changes.

What to Say

"The doctor said this could be a side effect of treatment. Let's call the infusion center and let them know what's going on."

"Maybe we should talk to a nutritionist about this, because what you eat and drink can make a difference."

"How about I take walks with you to help your body move through this [constipation]?"

"It's important that you rest when you are going through this [diarrhea]. How can I help decrease your stress level so you can focus on taking care of yourself?"

What to Do

- Listen empathetically and validate your loved one's feelings. Symptoms of diarrhea or constipation can be concerning and uncomfortable.

- Call the doctor/infusion center to report the symptoms. In the case of diarrhea, take your loved one's temperature and report that as well.

- For constipation, encourage the consumption of high-fiber foods and nonalcoholic fluids and increased exercise.

- For diarrhea, avoid greasy and fatty foods, dairy, and high-fiber or hard-to-digest foods like raw fruits and vegetables, beans, and whole grains.

- Watch for worrisome symptoms such as fever, pain, blood in stool, and nausea/vomiting, and report them to your loved one's medical team. With diarrhea, dehydration can occur, and you may need to take your loved one into the infusion center or emergency room for IV hydration.

- Assist by offering to do the grocery shopping and cooking and/or exercising with your loved one.

What to Ask Your Doctor

1. What diet do you recommend? What foods should be avoided?

2. What are some ways to add fiber to meals? Do you recommend fiber supplements?

3. What's a good daily goal for fluid intake?

4. What medications do you recommend?

5. For diarrhea, what are the things to watch for that would be a cause for concern?

6. Can you provide a referral to a dietician for support?

Nausea and Vomiting

Nausea and vomiting are two of the most dreaded side effects associated with cancer treatment. Fortunately, there are many antinausea/vomiting drugs that can help prevent and control symptoms. These medications, also known as antiemetics, can be given orally and intravenously before, during, and after chemotherapy. Some common antiemetics are Zofran (ondansetron), Compazine (prochlorperazine), lorazepam, and dexamethasone. Nausea and vomiting can also be mitigated through diet and other lifestyle habits.

What to Say

"Did you take your antinausea medications exactly as directed? If not, we should start that right away."

"You are doing everything as directed. Let's call the doctor/infusion center and see what they can do to help. We were told that nausea and vomiting should be well controlled through medication."

"I think there are some things we can do here at home that might help, like eating small meals and eating frequently throughout the day. If you allow yourself to get really hungry, it might make the nausea worse."

"I think you will learn what foods settle best with you. I can keep a journal so we can track that, if you'd like."

What to Do

- Be aware of the antinausea regimen prescribed to your loved one so you can make sure they are following the protocol.

- Report symptoms to the doctor/infusion center.

- Encourage nonalcoholic and noncaffeinated fluid intake, and provide fluids for your loved one. They may find it easier to drink through a straw.

- Be aware of greasy foods that may trigger nausea. Prepare food that can help prevent and control nausea, like dry cereal or toast.

- Keep the house free of strong odors such as perfumes, scented products, or any other items that are difficult for your loved one to tolerate.

- Keep fresh air flowing through the house. Encourage your loved one to spend time outdoors.

- Provide a calm and relaxing environment. It may be helpful to play soothing music. Let your loved one take the lead as to what makes them most comfortable.

What to Ask Your Doctor

1. Is the chemo regimen you are prescribing more likely to cause nausea/vomiting?

2. What medications will you prescribe to prevent and control nausea/vomiting?

3. Do those medications have side effects?

4. Is nausea more likely to occur during chemotherapy or afterward? Are there particularly difficult points in a chemo cycle?

5. If nausea is still a problem after following the protocol as prescribed, what do you recommend?

6. What red flags should we be aware of?

Pain

Pain is an unpleasant sensation that can vary greatly in severity. There are many different causes of pain, such as injury, illness, and certain medications and treatments. Cancer itself can cause pain when tumors invade the organs, bones, and nerves. Different treatments, such as surgery, chemotherapy, and radiation, may also cause pain. Whatever the cause, pain control is a high priority.

What to Say

"I want to help make you more comfortable."

"The doctor said you may have pain, but we should always report it. I will call now."

"I want to help report important information to the doctor about your pain. I have some questions to ask that may help the doctor better help you."

"I can imagine being in pain might make you feel down or irritable. I understand."

"I'm going to do everything I can to help get your pain under control. The oncologist said there is a palliative care doctor who can help with this. Would you like me to get us an appointment?"

What to Do

- Contact the doctor to report the pain and determine next steps.

- Offer to take on more responsibilities until the pain is better controlled.

- Be an advocate for your loved one. If pain isn't controlled with the prescriptions ordered, report that to the doctor.

- If needed, ask for a referral to a pain specialist or palliative care doctor.

- Help your loved one track their pain in terms of time, location, onset, severity, and what makes it better or worse. Use the pain scale (1 to 10, with 1 being the lowest).

- Encourage taking medications on a regular basis. Monitor this if your loved one is confused or forgetful.

- Notice signs of pain such as moaning, grimacing, or lack of movement.

- Try warm or cool compresses and light massage.

- Keep pain medications in a safe place.

- Encourage practices like yoga, meditation, biofeedback, acupuncture, and other forms of energy healing.

What to Ask Your Doctor

1. What can be done to better control pain?

2. What are the side effects of the pain medication you are prescribing?

3. Are there any negative interactions with other medications they are taking?

4. Are there any other tests needed to rule out other causes of the pain?

5. Are there any other providers that can help?

6. Getting a good night's rest is becoming difficult due to the pain. Is there anything you can prescribe for sleep?

7. Is addiction a concern with the prescribed medication?

8. What are your thoughts about cannabis for pain relief?

Sleep Problems

Sleep problems are common during cancer treatment. The emotional and physical stress of treatment, coupled with medication side effects, can wreak havoc on sleep. Getting adequate sleep, especially during treatment, is important for the healing process and for mental and emotional well-being. Let your doctor know if your loved one is experiencing insomnia. Depending on the cause, there may be a medication that can help or other guidelines to follow that can facilitate a better night's rest.

What to Say

"Not sleeping well is hard physically and emotionally. If you like, let's call the doctor to see if there are any medication options."

"Maybe some of your medications are causing sleep problems as a side effect. Let's ask the doctor about that."

"You must be tired from not sleeping well. I can take some things off your plate so you can get some rest."

"Sometimes people can't sleep because they have a lot on their mind. I am here to listen if you want to talk."

"After doing some research, I discovered tips for addressing sleep problems, such as increasing physical activity, making changes to your nighttime routine, and relaxation exercises."

What to Do

- Encourage talking with the doctor about medication options and to see if any currently prescribed medications can cause insomnia.

- Discuss good sleep hygiene, like turning off electronics a couple hours before bed, keeping the room dark, and trying to have a consistent sleep schedule.

- Suggest appropriate exercise, which can help combat insomnia and mood issues.

- Suggest cutting back on caffeine.

- If pain is not well controlled, contact the doctor.

- Beyond medical factors, explore other possible causes, such as anxiety and/or depression.

- Investigate alternative ways to combat stress, like yoga, meditation, deep breathing, acupuncture, or acupressure.

- Listen empathetically and validate your loved one's feelings.

What to Ask Your Doctor

1. Do you have any suggestions for addressing sleep problems?

2. Is there a medication that is safe to take, at least for a short time, in order to catch up on sleep a bit?

3. Are there any prescribed medications that might make sleep problems worse? If so, how long will they be needed? Are there any alternative medications with fewer sleep side effects?

When Treatment Ends

When cancer treatment ends, it is a time to celebrate and to recognize the cancer survivor's incredible strength and resilience. It is also when many cancer survivors ask, "Now that treatment is done, how do I want to spend my time, and with whom?" As they face mortality, many cancer survivors go inward and begin exploring what gives their life meaning. When treatment ends, they can feel catapulted into a new world, one they don't really recognize because they are no longer the same person. New priorities may arise, such as making a career change or shifting work hours. They may focus more on self-care and spending quality time with loved ones.

Although treatment can be a very difficult time, it provides a safe and structured environment where patients can actively fight the cancer. Afterward, some cancer survivors feel exposed and unstructured, and they may try to establish a "new normal." Many are afraid of the cancer returning and feel overwhelmed as they navigate the transition into survivorship. Without cancer treatment as the centerpiece of their life, they must create a new road map.

Thankfully, patients and caregivers have the support of the cancer team in the posttreatment phase as well. Programs vary in their scope of services, but many offer survivorship care plans, support groups, referrals to posttreatment nutrition and exercise programs, and integrative healing therapies that can all help ease the transition.

What to Say

"I understand you have a lot on your mind. It's going to take a little time to ease into this next phase."

"There are a lot of resources we can tap into as you move into this next phase. Would you like me to help you look into what's available?"

"My understanding is that people typically feel some side effects from treatment even after it's over. If you'd like, we can check in with the doctor just to make sure what you're experiencing is normal."

What to Do

- Follow your loved one's lead. Normalize and validate whatever feelings they have.
- Consult with the cancer support team to get educated about survivorship resources.
- Offer to attend follow-up appointments.

- Remind them that you are still there to support them.

- Assist with personal care or home-related tasks, running errands, and managing childcare, if applicable.

- Let your support network know they may still be needed and that your loved one's healing process will continue.

- Encourage continued self-care habits, such as good nutrition, exercise, and stress management.

What to Ask Your Doctor

1. Ask for a survivorship care plan? This summarizes the diagnosis and treatment history and specifies the recommended follow-up in terms of tests, lab work, and appointment intervals. Survivorship care plans also include information about staying healthy and provide resources and relevant referral information.

2. Clarify the process for posttreatment follow-up appointments? Will the office reach out to make appointments, or do you need to contact the office? If you need to contact the office, how long before the expected appointment date should you reach out? Some offices book far in advance. Be proactive.

How Are You Doing?

One of the greatest gifts caregivers can offer is walking alongside their loved one during treatment, hand in hand. Often a long and intense process, cancer treatment can take a physical and emotional toll on both survivors and caregivers. Caregiver fatigue can set in, and the need for self-care grows increasingly more important over time. Stress management practices, like this dia-phragmatic breathing exercise, can be helpful.

- Sit or lie down in a quiet, comfortable place. Be sure to bend your knees.
- Notice your breathing begins to slow as you bring your focus within yourself. Take a few long, deep breaths.
- Place one hand on your chest and one hand on your diaphragm. As you breathe in deeply and slowly, make a conscious effort to breathe from your diaphragm.
- Watch the hand on your diaphragm rise as you breathe in while the hand on your chest remains still.
- Thank your body for all that it does for you.
- Reflect on all you have done and given in your role.

CHAPTER 4

Common Daily Living Changes

JONAH

Jonah's father was diagnosed with a blood cancer at age 71, and his whole life shifted. "Before, my father did everything," Jonah remembers. "Almost immediately after his first treatment, it was clear his mental faculties were being affected, and it was like someone flipped a switch. This mountain of a man was crumbling, and I knew I had to do whatever was needed." Jonah immediately jumped in to assist his mother with overseeing his father's care, as well as the finances and household tasks. "My mom and I had to put on our internal MD hats. Initially, I felt like the best use of my time was to figure out what hospitals were doing cutting-edge research," he explains. Jonah traveled with his parents to every doctor's appointment, including those out of state at the Dana-Farber Cancer Institute. Together, Jonah and his mother assessed what was needed every step of the way and supported each other emotionally during difficult times. Jonah says, "I was shocked at the role change and how quickly it had to happen. When the people who are most important to you need you, you have to pull up your big boy pants, even if you don't feel ready." Jonah was involved in every aspect of his father's care, including daily personal care, transportation to appointments, and helping his mother. "I think being a father helped me," Jonah concludes. "I was already in a role of caring for my children and understood the responsibility."

Doctor's Appointments

Upon diagnosis, cancer survivors are faced with a great deal of stress and anxiety, along with the overwhelming responsibility of navigating the health-care system. Caregivers play a critical role in alleviating stress by becoming an integral member of the cancer care team. Taking on this role may include making appointments and providing vital advocacy as needed. Caregivers may also need to provide transportation to and from appointments, as well as take notes so that their loved one can focus on being present and truly listening to what the doctor is saying. Additionally, having another pair of eyes and ears at appointments can bring great comfort, as sometimes the doctor's words are complex and not always fully heard, questioned, or understood. Medical appointments can be frightening and traumatic, and having a loved one there provides greatly needed emotional support.

What to Say

"Would it be helpful if I accompanied you to your appointment? I would love to be a support."

"I'm going to bring a notepad so I can take notes. I want to free you up to listen to the doctor. I can also help remind you what you want to discuss."

"I want to be there to support you. I know going to the doctor can sometimes feel overwhelming, and having someone there to shoulder the load may be helpful."

"I think it will be helpful if I come with you to the doctor. Having two people listening is much better than one. That way things are less likely to be missed and we can be sure to ask everything you want to ask."

What to Do

- Help reduce stress by offering to coordinate care and make appointments. Interfacing with medical offices can be time-consuming and stressful.

- Help your loved one prepare a list of questions. Put them in order of importance.

- Ask how you can be most helpful regarding appointments. Would they like you to take notes, remind them of what they wish to ask, or provide emotional support?

- If seeing a new doctor, bring records and/or a medical history. Assist in procuring records as needed.

- Bring a comprehensive list of medications and supplements, or bring the actual bottles in a bag.

- During an appointment, try to let your loved one lead the conversation. Jump in if they need some support, but be careful not to take over the conversation.

- After appointments, offer your listening ear. Follow your loved one's lead as to whether they wish to talk or want your input.

What to Ask Your Doctor

1. For questions that come up after our visits, is it better to email you or call your office?

2. When will we be talking next? Will that be an in-person visit, a phone conversation, or email communication?

3. When reporting in, what information would be most helpful to share? It seems like more specifics would be better. Would you like a detailed description of symptoms, when they started, their severity, and what makes them better or worse? Please let me know what is most helpful for you to know.

4. Will you be communicating with other doctors on the team? Is there anything patients can do to help facilitate communication among their providers?

Eating and Nutrition

Cancer itself, as well as side effects from treatment, can lead to malnutrition. Some patients experience an increase or decrease in appetite, taste and smell changes, and other symptoms such as nausea, vomiting, diarrhea, constipation, and weight loss or gain. Some cannot eat or digest food normally and may have nutrient absorption problems.

Good nutrition plays a critical role in cancer care. It is a complex arena best navigated by a registered dietician with an expertise in oncology. They can design a nutrition program that specifically targets the unique needs of each patient through the different phases of treatment and into posttreatment. Dieticians are also available for fine-tuning the nutrition program and answering questions.

What to Say

"Maybe we can talk to an expert or dietician who can help us navigate this. If you like, I can look into finding one."

"I am here to support you if you want to make changes to your diet. I can help with the shopping and food preparation. Maybe we can get a good cookbook and make it fun."

What to Do

- Follow your loved one's lead. If you notice they are resistant to talking about nutrition, try not to push. Making lifestyle changes can be very difficult for some people, especially when they are already under emotional and physical stress.

- Should you feel overwhelmed by well-intentioned family or friends offering nutrition advice, gently tell them thank you, but that you prefer to get advice from a registered dietician with oncology expertise.

- When eating away from home or in restaurants, encourage your loved one to order their food the way they want it. If eating a big meal out together, consider eating smaller meals at home the remainder of the day.

- Encourage making changes in small increments. Increasing water intake, for example, can have tremendous health benefits and mitigate treatment side effects.

- Offer to help with shopping and food preparation.

What to Ask Your Doctor

1. During treatment, are there any special considerations regarding diet?

2. Can you provide a referral to a dietician for nutritional counseling?

3. Might any of the drugs in the treatment plan cause appetite changes? What suggestions do you have for managing this?

4. Who can review supplements to make sure they are okay to continue during treatment?

Family Communicator

Caregivers often find themselves assuming the role of primary communicator with family and friends. This responsibility can be both rewarding and stressful. Taking time to explain what is happening medically, as well as socially and emotionally, can feel therapeutic. Receiving loving and caring responses from the support network can be a comfort. On the other hand, fielding questions from well-meaning friends and family members can sometimes feel draining or frustrating. Although they may try, it can be very difficult for others to truly understand. Some suggestions may be very helpful and some may not. It is important that caregivers in the primary communicator role make their needs known in terms of both practical and emotional support. There may not be enough time and energy for individualized texts and emails. Sending out group communications can be a big time and energy saver. It is also a good idea to be clear about the best mode of communication for responses and offers of support.

What to Say

"If you would like, I would be happy to communicate with our support network, especially at times when you want to conserve some energy."

"Let's talk about what you would like me to communicate to our support network. What would you like them to know?"

"Let's go over some tasks we can delegate to our family and friends. They have asked how they can help."

"I know our family and friends mean well, but I have the sense that sometimes it feels overwhelming for you to talk to them. How can I help off-load this? We can talk about ways you can respond, or I can respond on your behalf."

What to Do

- Let your loved one know they don't have to shoulder all the communication on their own, and that you are there to help if needed.

- Sit down together to determine what information your loved one wishes to impart to their support network.

- Discuss websites that can facilitate communication and coordinate help. If your loved one is interested, you can offer to start a website or Facebook group.

- Together, determine what type of help would be useful, such as preparing meals, running errands, providing transportation and/or accompaniment to appointments, or assisting with childcare/playdates/pet care, when applicable.

- Offer to field inquiries from family and friends. Follow your loved one's lead as to how much or how little they want to be involved with communication.

- If well-meaning family and friends are saying and doing things your loved one finds challenging, offer to step in and share a better approach.

What to Ask Your Family and Friends

1. Be specific about what type of support is needed.

2. Encourage family and friends to listen, be supportive of whatever decisions are being made, and give advice only when asked.

3. Discourage sharing cancer stories that don't have a good ending.

4. Let family and friends know there may be times when you or your loved one don't want to talk about cancer. Suggest that they ask before jumping into the topic.

5. Set realistic expectations around communication. Let them know it might take some time to respond to their outreach due to the demands of treatment. Although there will be instances when visits are welcome, communicate the need to decline visits or set time limits depending on your loved one's energy level.

Medication

At times, a caregiver may need to assist with administering medications in the form of pills, liquids, or injections. It is critical to take the right medication at the right time and extremely important to be aware of drug interactions. The learning curve can feel steep initially as you learn about the different medications, their dosages, and how and when to give them. It is important to connect with providers at the oncology clinic and the oncology pharmacists so you can learn the protocols and receive hands-on training as needed. If home health or hospice nurses are coming to the home, they can explain medication administration at the bedside.

There are a variety of tools that can be helpful with administering medications. Pill organizers let you divide up medications according to day and time and can be set up for a week at a time. Additional tools include pill dispensers, alarm-style reminders, and timer medicine caps.

What to Say

"It may be best at this point for me to start helping you with your medications. It's a lot to keep track of, and I wouldn't want you to miss any doses."

"The doctor said, for safety reasons, it would be best if I take over giving you your medications. They explained everything I need to do, and I am confident it will all go well."

"I have written down all your medications and understand the doses and when you need them. I also know what the possible side effects are and when to call the doctor."

"I got something to help us keep track of your medications [such as a pill organizer]."

What to Do

- Get educated on all the medications prescribed. Read the labels and take note of the name of each medication, the dosage, and the directions for use. Learn the side effects so you can help recognize problems early on and report them to the doctor.

- If your loved one has been administering their own medications, keep a watchful eye. If you are concerned that they are growing weaker or their mental status is changing, begin overseeing the process.

- Set up a pill organizer and keep it out of sight. Be present when it's time to give medications so you can be sure it gets done correctly.

- Be sure your loved one swallows all medications. If there are challenges with swallowing, ask the doctor if the medication can be given in another form, such as a liquid.

- If you need to administer injections, be sure to get proper training from the oncology staff.

1. At what point is it clear that medication assistance is needed?

2. What tools do you recommend to organize medications (such as a pill organizer)?

3. Doing self-injections is a bit scary. Is it okay for someone else to do them, and if so, what training is available?

4. What if there comes a point when medications can no longer be swallowed? Are there other options for how to ingest them?

5. Can you or someone in your office provide a list of all the medications, dosages, and directions for use?

Staying Active

Research indicates that staying physically active both during and after cancer treatment can help alleviate treatment side effects and improve quality of life. While getting enough rest during treatment is extremely important, it is equally important to keep moving. Movement can help improve mood and sleep, decrease anxiety and pain, and increase energy.

Those undergoing treatment should get clearance from their doctor before starting an exercise program. The recommended guidelines are 75 to 150 minutes of exercise per week, as tolerated. If that is not attainable, any kind of movement for any length of time is still beneficial. Gentle stretching and walking are good places to start. When ready, your loved one can work toward a combination of resistance training (such as weightlifting or exercises involving resistance bands), stretching and balance exercises, and cardio (such as walking, jogging, bicycling, or dance).

Treatment can cause side effects such as fatigue that may make it difficult for the patient to want to move. They should start slowly and observe how much movement their body can handle from day to day.

What to Say

"Would you like to go for a walk together? It might be nice to get some fresh air and movement. I can do this regularly with you if that would help motivate you to get out."

"I can imagine you are feeling tired, which makes it harder to want to be physically active. I think you may feel better after doing even a little movement, like walking around the house or doing some gentle stretching."

"I remember the cancer care coordinator told us there is an exercise program specifically for cancer survivors. I can get the details if you'd like, and maybe you can consider joining."

What to Do

- Meet your loved one where they are. Make gentle suggestions on how they can incorporate movement into their life, but try to avoid pushing or being overbearing.

- Offer to join in activities such as going to the gym, doing an online exercise class, and walking. If possible, walk or hike in nature. Many find this activity healing on all levels.

- Ask the cancer care coordinator if there are any local exercise programs specifically geared toward cancer recovery. Some cancer centers offer exercise classes in-house. People sometimes feel more motivated in a group setting.

- Encourage a daily routine when energy permits. Encourage exercising in small increments so the body has time to adjust before it is asked to do more.

- Think of ways to make movement fun. Perhaps suggest a walk around town coupled with a stop at a local restaurant or coffee house.

- Talk about all the ways exercise can help, such as by mitigating treatment side effects, maintaining weight, and boosting the immune system.

What to Ask Your Doctor

1. At what point can physical activity be resumed?

2. Are there any limitations as to what activities can be done?

3. What type of physical activity do you recommend?

4. Are there any times that exercise should be avoided?

5. Are you aware of any exercise programs for cancer survivors?

6. Should exercise in public places be avoided?

7. Would physical therapy be helpful in this case?

Personal Hygiene

People undergoing cancer treatment sometimes reach a point when they need assistance with personal care. For many caregivers, this is a new experience, and it can take time to learn how to integrate it into the daily routine. It calls on both caregivers and their loved ones to adapt to changes in how they relate to one another. For some, it may bring up some tension and discomfort, especially if your loved one is particularly modest or private.

There are many resources available that provide information on and training in personal care, including websites and online training courses. If caregivers cannot manage the responsibility on their own, it may be necessary to hire a private-duty caregiver. Your cancer care team can provide information and resources if you choose to pursue that option.

What to Say

"This is new for both of us. I want to follow your lead as to what I can do to be of help."

"What are you finding difficult to do on your own? I can help make things easier."

"Please be sure to tell me if something in this process makes you uncomfortable. I am learning and would really appreciate the feedback."

"Now that we're doing this together, I want you to feel free to tell me how you like things done, from how warm you like your water temperature to what lotions or products you like best and the way you style your hair."

What to Do

- Provide opportunities for your loved one to express how they feel about needing help with personal care. Actively listen and validate their feelings.

- Allow them to maintain as much independence as possible and encourage them to stay engaged.

- Do what you can to create a peaceful environment, such as by lowering the lights and putting on soft music.

- Find out what's best regarding time of day and frequency of personal care visits. Establish a routine.

- An occupational therapist (OT) can help modify the home so your loved one can stay independent longer. They can also address any safety concerns and adjust equipment.

- Investigate hygiene aids, such as shower chairs and long-handled shower brushes, that can make personal care easier.

- If needed and within your budget, consider hiring a professional caregiver. Ask the doctor's office or cancer care coordinator for resource information on private-duty caregivers.

What to Ask Your Doctor

1. I know treatment can increase risk of infection. Is there any personal care that should be avoided during treatment due to this risk?

2. Personal care is getting more difficult. Can you help determine what is still safe to do independently and what requires assistance?

3. At what point do people consider hiring help?

4. Are there any in-home services available, such as an aide, physical therapist, or occupational therapist?

5. What equipment can be ordered to make things easier at home, such as a shower chair or raised toilet seat?

Safety at Home

One of a caregiver's highest priorities is their loved one's safety. When someone grows weaker and is less able to care for themselves, home safety concerns can arise. The risk of falls and other injuries can greatly increase, and fires can result from misuse of the stove.

Many interventions can enhance safety in the home. An occupational therapist or in-home care aide can do a home safety assessment, making recommendations and providing resource information. Increasing in-home support through the help of family, friends, and/or private-duty caregivers may be necessary as well. Installing a medical alert system, bringing in medical equipment to aid in mobility and daily personal care, and making the space free of hazards and slippery surfaces can also help mitigate risk.

What to Say

"I noticed that you are a bit unsteady on your feet. Let's talk about some things we can do to help prevent a fall."

"I want to support you in being independent as long as possible. At the same time, I want to ensure you are safe."

"There are professionals that can come to the house and give us ideas on how to make it safer. Would it be okay with you if I look into that?"

"I'm wondering how you would feel about having a caregiver come in a couple days a week to help with things here. It might take some of the burden off of you."

What to Do

- Contact the doctor about a referral for a home safety assessment.

- Check your loved one's insurance to see what coverage exists for durable medical equipment, such as mobility devices (like walkers), grab bars, raised toilet seats, and shower chairs. If insurance does not cover an item(s), check local medical supply stores.

- Remove all fall hazards, such as slippery throw rugs. Clear space so there is plenty of room for moving around, especially if your loved one is using a walker or wheelchair.

- Consider getting a medical alert system.

- Keep emergency numbers in a visible, easy-to-reach place.

- Protect against fire by changing batteries regularly in smoke and carbon monoxide detectors and removing fire hazards like candles.

What to Ask Your Doctor

1. When weakness increases and falls and injuries are more likely, what suggestions do you have for home safety?

2. Can you provide a referral for an occupational therapist to come and do a safety assessment?

3. Based on your assessment, do you think more in-home support is needed?

4. What do you think of medical alert systems? Is there one that you recommend over others?

5. What about equipment for the house? Do you recommend anything that would help make the house safer and prevent falls and other injuries?

Schedules and Transportation

During cancer care, managing schedules and transportation needs can be challenging. Some treatment regimens require frequent visits to the clinic; radiation therapy, for example, is typically done on a daily basis for a specified period. For those who live a long distance from treatment, access can be difficult. There may be times when a loved one is no longer able to drive. Then, caregivers must step in and mobilize the support network to bridge the gaps. Utilize friends and family members who have graciously offered their support. Community transportation resources, such as the American Cancer Society's Road to Recovery program, can also provide rides to and from appointments. Many communities provide transportation for those considered too disabled to ride public transportation, which may include door-to-door service and shared rides. Your cancer care coordinator can connect you with these resources. Be aware that many require an application process.

What to Say

"I will feel better if someone takes you to your appointments since you are feeling tired and may have a reaction to the treatments."

"I'm going to talk to the cancer care coordinator about what resources are available for transportation and get you signed up. Without that worry, you can focus on your healing."

"I think transportation is going to be a big need. I will put the word out and get a schedule going."

What to Do

- Ask your provider for a treatment schedule indicating appointment dates and times.

- Reach out to your support network and let them know that you will have transportation needs. Be as specific as possible about dates and times.

- Contact the American Cancer Society in your area and register for the Road to Recovery program. Because it is a volunteer-run program, rides are not guaranteed, so it's important to have a backup plan should a ride fall through.

- Arrange backup transportation, such as Uber, Lyft, or local transportation services for the disabled, which may provide door-to-door service and shared rides.

- Consider registering on a website that helps organize assistance, such as CaringBridge.org or LotsaHelpingHands.com.

Sex and Intimacy

Cancer's impact on intimate relationships can be both positive and challenging. Although going through cancer can bring couples closer in many ways, it can also put a strain on sex and intimacy. Both cancer and cancer treatments can cause physical, mental, and emotional changes that may make sexual intimacy more difficult. Erectile dysfunction, vaginal dryness, fatigue, hormonal changes, nausea, pain, anxiety, and depression can alter sexual functioning and desire. Physical appearance can change and may affect self-image. For couples, this can be a difficult road to navigate, but talking openly with one another about the impact of cancer on your intimate life can allow you to work through it together.

Seek information and guidance from your doctor. Connecting with a mental health professional for advice can also be beneficial. A support group can offer a safe place to share with others who may be in similar situations. In addition, it is important to be aware that some sexual activity can be unsafe if practiced during certain periods of treatment. Those undergoing chemotherapy are particularly immunocompromised when their blood counts are low, and sexual intercourse and oral-genital stimulation are not advised at those times due to risk of infection. Do not have unprotected sex during treatment, as the chemotherapy could adversely affect your partner. For those that can get pregnant, it is critical to use birth control because chemotherapy could cause birth defects.

What to Say

"I love you and want you to know I am here to support you and listen."

"We are a team, and I am in this with you."

"I don't need to have sex to feel close to you. I love being with you and spending time together."

"I know this is a time for you to heal and recover and that you may not feel like having sex or being intimate. I understand."

"There are many ways to be intimate. We may just need some guidance. Maybe we should talk to the doctor or see a counselor to discuss ways we can stay close."

What to Do

- Provide a safe space for your loved one to talk about their concerns and for you to share yours.

- Offer compliments. Going through cancer can cause changes in appearance and self-image. It is important that your loved one knows you still find them attractive.

- Assure your loved one you are there for them and will be by their side for the duration of this experience.

- If having a third party to talk with would be helpful, get a referral to a good therapist with oncology expertise or a sex therapist.

- Consider joining a support group (individually or together) to talk about your concerns with people who are facing similar challenges.

- Carve out time for intimacy through activities such as dates and outings, as well as quiet time at home.

- Go slowly and follow your loved one's lead. Some days may be better than others in terms of your partner's sexual desire and energy during treatment.

What to Ask Your Doctor

1. Is it okay to have sex while in treatment? Is protection advised?

2. Are there times during treatment when it's better not to have sex?

3. What recommendations do you have for dealing with sexual side effects from treatment?

4. What effect does treatment have on fertility? If someone wants to preserve fertility, what is the process? Can you provide a referral for more information?

5. Can you recommend any remedies for pain with intercourse?

6. Can you recommend a professional who can help us with this?

How Are You Doing?

A caregiver's journey flows like a river: sometimes calmly and sometimes wildly. Caregivers may be asked to wear many hats simultaneously, juggling competing roles as researcher, organizer, advocate, communicator, delegator, and listener.

One way to help manage the stress is to become more mindful about time management. With so many important tasks to accomplish, it may be difficult to know how to prioritize your time.

Here are a few tips to help guide you:

- Each day, prioritize your to-do list. Ask yourself what needs immediate attention.
- Delegate tasks that do not require your involvement to your support network.
- Maintain a schedule. Use a calendar or some other organizer to track appointments and other important events.
- Set aside time to go to the gym, attend a support group, or meet up with a friend.
- Set goals to accomplish. For example, you may want to get some legal and financial documents in order. List this as one of your goals and set a timeline for it.
- Try to stay organized and plan ahead.

CHAPTER 5

Financial and Legal Decisions

APOLLO

Apollo's mother, Zoe, age 79, was diagnosed with stage IV bladder cancer. Apollo was no stranger to caregiving, having cared for Zoe since she had fallen and injured her head six years prior. In caring for Zoe, Apollo learned firsthand the importance of being prepared when it came to legal and financial issues. "Thankfully, my mother had already arranged a trust and a health-care directive naming me and my sister as her decision makers," Apollo says. After months recovering in the ICU and rehabilitation facilities, Zoe was finally able to go home, but her family needed to quickly determine how to meet her caregiving needs. "My parents had some savings and they took a second mortgage on the house, so we were able to hire caregivers," Apollo explains. He and his sister took turns visiting and divided up responsibilities, pitching in financially to help cover care costs. Several years later, Apollo and his sister were able to move their parents closer to where they live. "Before," he says, "my mother wasn't able to go outside because we couldn't get the wheelchair down the stairs. Now, she can enjoy the garden and fresh air. Her smile just lights up the room." Since their funds no longer support outside caregiving help, Apollo, his sister, their respective spouses, and hospice are now sharing the 24/7 caregiving responsibilities: "Between all of us, we are so blessed to have everyone coming together, able to make decisions, all one core unit trying to make it better."

Finances

When someone is diagnosed with cancer, one of the immediate areas of concern is often money. Caregiving needs and their associated costs can vary greatly depending on the type and length of treatment, the patient's previous level of functioning, and the extent to which family and friends can aid in the caregiving process. Many cancer survivors can maintain independence during treatment, but others need more regular, hands-on help. Time affords some the ability to plan for the future. However, for those diagnosed at a more advanced stage or experiencing debilitating symptoms, there may be an urgent need to mobilize an effective caregiving plan and financial approach.

Financial stress can be one of the most challenging aspects of a cancer diagnosis. Patients and caregivers may lose income if they cannot work or must work less due to treatment demands. There will likely be an increase in medical bills, including co-pay and deductible expenses. There may also be additional costs like private-duty caregiving, which can average anywhere from $15 to $30 per hour. For those who need long-term care placement, assisted living or nursing home costs range widely, landing in the thousands per month.

Just as treatments for different illnesses vary, so do the ways people approach financial management. Some stay in the present, thinking about immediate needs, whereas others prefer to plan ahead and anticipate financial needs. Whatever your unique situation, there are valuable resources available to assist you.

If you are experiencing financial stress, start by contacting your cancer care coordinator to discuss available resources. To help deal with income loss, your loved one may qualify for employee benefits, such as sick time, paid time off (PTO), or short-term state disability. Inquire about community resources that provide assistance, like home-delivered meals and emergency funding for rent or mortgage payments, medical costs, and other critical expenses. Medicaid provides health insurance coverage for those who meet the financial and medical eligibility requirements and can also help offset caregiving expenses. (See page 99 for more on Medicaid.)

Other potential resources to investigate include Social Security benefits and retirement accounts, such as 401(k) plans and pensions. You can start collecting Social Security as early as age 62, and some retirement accounts can be accessed early if needed. However, keep in mind that there may be reduced benefits or penalties for tapping into these funds early. If your loved one has taken out long-term care insurance, contact the company and thoroughly investigate what the policy offers and what is required to initiate the benefits. Review the fine print, as there may be exclusions and stipulations.

Consider developing a financial plan, either with a professional or on your own. Determining household income and assets, establishing a budget, and prioritizing expenses are the building blocks of a good financial plan. Should you wish to use a financial planner, ask your cancer care team if they know of any resources. Some financial planners provide pro bono services to people with cancer who cannot otherwise afford them. Interview potential candidates about their experience with costs associated with cancer. Take inventory of the areas that are important to you, such as medical coverage and disability, and be sure your candidate has expertise in them.

Finally, some may look to fundraising, such as GoFundMe campaigns, as a resource to help manage expenses.

What to Say

"I can imagine this feels stressful, and I am going to help you. Let's start by making a list of all of our questions."

"There is so much to consider, and I don't want to miss anything. I will start asking around for a referral for a financial advisor."

"I think the cancer care coordinator will help us figure out where to start and connect us with some resources."

"We need to start pulling some documents together. I may need your help, but I'll do as much as I can."

What to Do

- Make a list of your questions and concerns. Put them in order of importance so you know what to tackle first.

- Connect with the cancer care coordinator. Be open to hearing about any and all resources available. Share your questions and concerns.

- If you and/or your loved one are employed, contact your employer's human resources department to discuss income sources such as sick time, paid time off, and short-term disability (applicable to patients only).

- Gather bank statements, investment portfolio documents, and any retirement or HSA (health savings account) documents. Take an inventory of all income sources, assets, and debts.

- Make a monthly budget that allows for increased medical and caregiving expenses.

- Ask friends, family, and professionals you know, such as lawyers or accountants, for financial planner referrals.

- Medicaid can provide funding for in-home caregiving support and long-term care. Familiarize yourself with the eligibility criteria and apply if you qualify.

What to Ask Your Financial Advisor

1. Do you have expertise that may be beneficial to cancer survivors, such as knowledge of disability benefits, medical coverage, and life insurance?

2. What documents do you need to create a financial plan?

3. What information do you need to help create a budget?

4. What are your fees? Do you charge by the hour or by the project, or do you incorporate fees into investments?

5. How long have you been in the business?

6. Can you provide references?

7. Are you familiar with domestic partnerships and how they differ from legal marriage, as well as any relevant tax implications?

8. How can we ensure there are some financial resources left for surviving family members in the event of a death?

Insurance

The world of health insurance is complex, and navigating it requires time, energy, and a strategy. Some people are very fortunate to have comprehensive coverage and small out-of-pocket expenses. Others may be uninsured or underinsured, carrying policies with high deductibles, co-pays, and coinsurance. Your cancer care coordinator can help provide some direction.

Patients who are uninsured can speak with their medical center's administrative offices about the available health coverage options and how to approach the application process. Some may qualify for their state's Medicaid program, which requires certain medical and financial criteria be met. Inquire with your medical center to see if they offer assistance with the Medicaid application process. If they don't, look up Medicaid in your state and find the closest office's address and phone number. The application process varies from state to state and may be possible to complete online and/or in-person. You may also consider the Health Insurance Marketplace under the Affordable Care Act (ACA), which provides access to health insurance at a more affordable cost for those who qualify. The ACA ensures that you cannot be denied coverage based on pre-existing conditions. You can find information online at Healthcare. gov. You can also contact an insurance agent who specializes in health care at no charge. They can assist in navigating the vast array of policies available. Be cautious when choosing a policy. Make sure you understand the coverage thoroughly, including the cost of the premium, deductible, co-pays, and coinsurance, which is the percentage of the cost of services that is your responsibility.

If your loved one has health-care coverage, call the insurance company's customer service department and go through the plan coverage carefully. If you anticipate that the financial burden may become unmanageable, contact your medical center's billing department, as many offer a payment plan option. There may also be a patient assistance program that can reduce or eliminate out-of-pocket costs for a period of time. An application is typically required. Eligibility is determined based on financial need and may require submission of recent tax returns, pay stubs, and bank statements.

Many organizations also have "cancer funds" that provide cash assistance for housing, food, medical bills, and other essential expenses. The American Cancer Society has an extensive national database of programs and organizations that support cancer survivors and their loved ones. Your cancer care coordinator may also have knowledge of such programs.

If someone loses insurance coverage during cancer treatment because they leave their job, there may be an option to maintain the same plan for a specified period under COBRA (Consolidated Omnibus Budget Reconciliation Act). Their former company's human resources department can provide information on COBRA options.

To save money on drugs, talk with your doctors to ensure they are ordering only what is necessary at the appropriate intervals. Consider patient assistance programs such as GoodRx (GoodRx. com), a website that provides cost comparisons among pharmacies and help finding manufacturer discount coupons and savings programs. These programs can make prohibitively expensive drugs more affordable for those who financially qualify. You can also find information about these programs on drug manufacturer websites.

What to Say

"I want to learn about our health coverage in detail so we can plan for additional medical expenses. We can do it together, but if you don't feel up to it, I can make that call on my own."

"There are some options for getting coverage. I'm going to talk to the cancer care coordinator so I can get some direction."

"I know these bills coming in are stressful. I'm going to contact the billing department to see if we can be put on a payment plan and consolidate everything into one manageable payment every month."

What to Do

- Contact the cancer care coordinator about available resources.

- If uninsured, determine if the medical facility has a business office that can assist you in applying for coverage.

- Investigate all avenues of possible coverage and any policies that an insurance agent recommends.

- Find out all policy details before committing. Be certain the plan will cover a diagnosis of cancer, and determine out-of-pocket expenses, including the premium, co-pays, coinsurance, and deductibles.

- If insured, call the insurance company and go over the policy in detail with a customer service representative. Discuss what is and is not covered, what services require a co-pay and the cost, any coinsurance requirements, and the maximum out-of-pocket expenditure for the year.

- Ask the cancer care coordinator if the medical center offers a patient assistance program that may reduce or eliminate out-of-pocket charges for a period of time.

- Establish a contact at your center's billing department. Ask if they offer a payment plan and what it entails.

What to Ask Your Insurance Provider

1. My loved one was just diagnosed with cancer. What medical services are not covered by the plan?

2. What percentage does the plan pay after meeting the deductible?

3. Are there any medical services that are not subject to the deductible?

4. What are the co-pay costs for each service, including office visits, laboratory work, diagnostic testing, emergency room visits, and procedures?

5. What is the coinsurance percentage for a hospital stay? What other services are subject to coinsurance?

6. Can you send me anything in writing that provides an overview of the coverage and is easy to follow and understand?

Legal Matters

Addressing legal matters is an important component of developing a comprehensive cancer care plan. Executing legal documents that explicitly state one's wishes and who will carry them out brings clarity and peace of mind and provides emotional and financial protections for survivors and their loved ones.

All of the following documents and instructions for execution can be found online. You can also consult an attorney and your cancer care coordinator for assistance.

A *Durable Power of Attorney for Health Care (DPAHC)* appoints and authorizes someone to make health-care decisions on behalf of the patient should the patient no longer be capable of making their own decisions. Some medical centers have staff in place to help facilitate the process of executing a DPAHC. More than one decision maker (sometimes called a "health-care agent") can be appointed. Although the document itself is important, of equal or greater importance is determining what the patient's wishes are and communicating them to the appointed decision maker(s).

A *living will* differs from a DPAHC in that it is specific to end-of-life health-care decisions (whereas the DPAHC covers all medical circumstances). Many people choose to have both a DPAHC and a living will. Together or separately, these documents ensure that a trusted person(s) is able to carry out the patient's wishes and prevent unwanted court involvement.

A *Power of Attorney for Finances* appoints someone to carry out financial decision-making should the patient no longer have the capacity to do so. This document can vary in scope, granting a range of powers like making payments, handling the buying and selling of property, and managing investment accounts.

A *will* is an estate-planning document that outlines how a person wishes their estate to be distributed after their death. If children are involved, it can specify guardianship. It also names the executor of the estate, who carries out the wishes outlined in the will. A will goes through probate court, a process by which a person's estate is reconciled prior to the distribution of property to beneficiaries. This can be a lengthy and costly process due to court and attorney fees. If you die without a will, the destiny of your estate and guardianship of minor children will be determined based upon the laws of your state.

A *trust* is different from a will. A will becomes active at the time of death, whereas a trust becomes active at the time the document is executed. One of the primary reasons people create a trust is to avoid probate court. There are different types of trusts, with advantages and disadvantages to each. Although there are "do-it-yourself" trusts online, it may be prudent to contact an attorney if the estate is large or complex or if the prospect of creating a trust feels overwhelming or uncomfortable for you or your loved one.

What to Say

"I think planning for the future is important, and I am learning that there are some legal documents we can get in order to help put our minds at ease."

"We may someday be in a position where we can't make our own health-care decisions. There's a form we can both fill out to legally appoint someone to make decisions for us if we cannot for ourselves. We can do this together."

"This might be a good time to start thinking about putting our affairs in order so you don't have to worry about it later on. Maybe we can seek out a lawyer who can help us with this. I'm happy to make some calls."

What to Do

- Ask your cancer care coordinator about any resources.

- Find out what existing legal documents your loved one may have already completed. Locate and update any existing documents. Make sure copies of documents are distributed to all the important parties. For example, the Durable Power of Attorney for Health Care needs to be given to the hospital/medical center and medical decision makers. A copy will also be kept in the medical chart.

- If legal matters have not yet been addressed, open the dialogue gently and with compassion. Offer to talk about their wishes in both the medical and financial arenas.

- If finances permit, consider hiring a licensed estate attorney. The attorney can answer questions, guide you through the process, and execute the documents.

- For concerns about workplace discrimination, search for information online about the Americans with Disabilities Act (ADA). Consider consulting with an employment attorney.

What to Ask Your Lawyer

1. What legal documents do you recommend we execute?

2. What information do you need to draft these documents?

3. How much will it cost to complete the estate plan?

4. What are the pros and cons of establishing a trust?

5. I have heard there are different types of trusts. What do you recommend in this situation?

6. Do you recommend having both a will and a trust?

How Are You Doing?

Handling financial and legal matters can be stressful even in the best of times. If you discover that your overwhelmed loved one needs advocacy, take a moment to acknowledge how invaluable your assistance is. Remember how much you are off-loading for your loved one by taking over these vital reins. Most important, turn inward for a few moments and focus on your own well-being. Are you getting enough rest and adequate sleep to face the demands of your caregiving role?

Good sleep practices, also known as sleep hygiene, can improve the quality and quantity of your sleep. Here are some suggestions for getting a better night's rest:

- Get on a consistent sleep schedule by going to bed and waking up around the same time every day.
- Establish a pre-bedtime routine. Consider a relaxation practice such as yoga/stretching, breathing exercises, meditation, or taking a warm bath/shower.
- Avoid caffeine, alcohol, and nicotine for four to six hours before bedtime.
- Make your bedroom a sleep sanctuary. Keep it at your preferred temperature, dark, and quiet.
- Have a cutoff time for watching TV and using your phone and computer, preferably one to two hours before bed.
- Avoid eating and exercising late in the day. Try to begin settling down at least three hours before bedtime.
- If you nap, try doing it earlier in the day. Naps too close to bedtime can interfere with sleep.

CHAPTER 6

Long-Term Caregiving Help

ANITA

Anita was diagnosed at the age of 77 with lung cancer that had metasta-sized to the brain. She lived alone and initially was able to take good care of herself and maintain independence. Her daughter, Kim, an only child, lived close by and assisted as needed. With time, Anita became weaker, and the cancer started to affect her memory and daily functioning.

Although Kim worked full time, she was able to step in and take over more responsibilities. "It was really hard," she recalls, "but I was determined to keep my mother in her home for as long as possible." Over time, Kim became increasingly concerned about her mother's safety and knew she needed to hire some help. Although their financial resources were limited, they covered a caregiver for a few hours a day, but eventu-ally it became clear that Anita needed 24-hour help.

"This was a very stressful point because we could only afford a few months in assisted living and I knew I had to come up with a feasible plan for long-term care," Kim explains. She found an assisted living facility and simultaneously looked into nursing home options. She educated herself about financing long-term care and consulted with a Medicaid specialist who helped her with the application process. Kim looked at many nursing homes and found one that accepted Medicaid. She felt it was a good decision: "I knew that my mother would be in a safe place and get good care. For me, that was what was most important."

Getting Additional Caregiving Help

Caregivers and their loved ones often grapple with the idea of hiring outside help. It can be hard to recognize when it's time to do so. Caregivers get so used to a high level of stress, they may miss the warning signs of burnout, which can put their own physical and emotional health in jeopardy. Caregiver stress can manifest in exhaustion, poor sleep, weight gain or loss, substance abuse, and emotions like anger, frustration, irritability, hopelessness, and depression. Sometimes, it takes an outside person like another family member or friend to gently point out the need for additional support.

At times, it is the patient who is reluctant to accept outside help, perhaps because they are private and find it difficult to build trust with someone they don't know. If your loved one adamantly refuses much-needed hired help, here are some strategies that can help them feel more comfortable with the idea:

- Get clear about what help is truly needed versus what would be nice to have. Focus only on that which is necessary for the safety and well-being of your loved one.
- Listen to your loved one's concerns. Determine what the underlying issues are, such as a fear of loss of independence.
- Show empathy and validate their feelings. Try not to get into a power struggle. Highlight all the positive aspects of their lives and what they are able to manage on their own.
- Start in small increments. Even if you need someone several hours daily, begin the conversation by suggesting two hours a day for one or two days per week.
- Introduce the caregiver in a nonthreatening manner, such as by going on a walk together or sitting and enjoying coffee or tea.
- Help your loved one feel like part of the process by interviewing candidates together. Take their input in determining the caregiver's hours, days, and duties.

- Consider having a doctor, nurse, social worker, or friend broach the topic. Sometimes hearing the suggestion from an outside source takes the charge or stigma out of it.
- Be honest. If you can no longer manage the caregiving on your own and your loved one's safety and well-being are compromised, state that clearly. They may be more open to the help if they understand it is for you as much as it is for them.
- If you remain at an impasse after trying these strategies, you may need to allow the situation to unfold as it will. Continue to offer support, and if your loved one has a change of heart, you will be ready to implement the plan.

First, determine whether the need is for skilled care or custodial (nonmedical) care. Skilled care refers to care that is provided by someone with a license or certification, such as a nurse, home health aide, social worker, or physical/occupational therapist. Custodial care refers to assistance with bathing, dressing, meal preparation, errands, and supervision and can be done by anyone with caregiving skills. Your loved one's doctor is the best person to help determine what type of care is needed. If the doctor believes home health care is needed and the criteria for referral are met, they will order the care and direct you on how to connect with a home care agency. Although many insurance plans cover home health care, some do not. Home care agencies can run a benefits check to see if your insurance will cover their services.

For custodial care services, you can use an agency that provides caregivers or you can hire someone independently. There are significant differences between these two options. Agency charges range from $20 to $30 per hour on average, and pricing varies by geography. The caregiver is employed by the agency. The cost of independently hired caregivers is about $10 to $20 per hour, and the caregiver is considered a household employee. Agencies handle the vetting process, insurance, and scheduling, whereas these responsibilities fall to the patient and caregiver in an independent hire situation. Live-in caregiver costs range widely, from about $1,000 to $5,000 per month.

For those with Medicaid benefits (see page 99), the cost of in-home caregiving *may* be partially or fully covered. If your loved one has Medicaid, contact your local Medicaid office for further information. Please note: Medicare *does not* cover in-home care-givers, aside from home health-care services ordered by a doctor.

What to Say

"It might be time to consider hiring someone to come in and help. As much as I want to be able to do everything for you, I'm no longer able to manage it all on my own."

"Having someone come to help out will allow you to maintain your independence."

"I know cooking and cleaning are not your favorite activities. How about we have someone come in to do those tasks so you can focus on the things you enjoy?"

"Your safety is what's most important. Having someone here a bit more often would put everyone's mind at ease."

What to Do

- Check to see if your loved one has a long-term care policy that includes home help coverage.

- Talk to the doctor to see if home health care is appropriate. If so, follow up closely to be sure home health care has been ordered. Determine which agency you would like to use, and be sure their services are covered by insur-ance. Ask the cancer care team, friends, and family for recommendations.

- Assess home care needs like supervision, housecleaning, meal prep, or personal care.

- Speak with your loved one about the care in a gentle, compassionate manner.

- Check your budget to see what money is available for caregiving help.

- If your loved one has limited resources, consider applying for Medicaid.

- If you are hiring a caregiver independently, seek out trustworthy sources and thoroughly check all references. Strongly consider contacting a certified public accountant (CPA) for assistance with setting up payroll and understanding the rules and responsibilities of household employment, including any relevant tax implications.

What to Ask a Service Provider

1. What services will you be providing? Are there multiple people involved?

2. Is this covered by insurance or are there out-of-pocket costs?

3. How many times per week do you recommend visits?

4. How do you gain the trust of the people you work with?

5. Can you recommend a way to explain to my loved one why these services are needed?

6. Will you be offering an introductory visit to explain the services to my loved one?

Long-Term Care

There may come a point when you need to consider long-term care. A variety of situations can precipitate this consideration, including the following:

- Caregiving needs cannot be met in an independent living environment.
- There are overarching medical needs that require a higher level of care.
- It is cost prohibitive to fund private-duty caregivers in the home setting.
- Independent living may have become too isolating, and long-term care provides social interaction and activities.

It is important to explore the many long-term care options available. For some, making this transition feels like a natural next step when it is clear they need the help and support. For others, it can be met by harsh resistance and a strong, stubborn desire to remain independent. Each individual's reaction is completely valid and understandable.

In some cultures, it is the norm for families to care for their elders in the home rather than seek long-term care placement. Many families live in multigenerational households where each generation is valued for its contributions to the family system. Cultural norms are passed down through the generations, and children grow up with the understanding that as their parents age, the family will strive to come together to provide care.

Caregivers who are in the position of seeking long-term care for their loved one need information and support. Ideally, the process can take place over time so there is room to gather information and thoroughly consider all options. The first step to obtaining any kind of caregiving help, whether in-home or in a facility, is to perform a financial assessment to see what resources are available. Some people have already made arrangements by purchasing long-term care insurance and possibly enlisting a financial planner to help ensure that funds are available for long-term care. Others may need to start by learning about the primary options for long-term care, some of which are listed here.

Assisted living describes a wide range of living environments. Residents typically have their own living space and venture out for meals and other activities. The common thread between these environments is the provision of help with daily living tasks. Some assisted living facilities offer meals and minimal in-home care, whereas others may offer a full range of care services. The cost of assisted living varies greatly based on geography, the level of care offered, and amenities, with a range from about $2,500 to $5,500 per month. Medicare does *not* cover the cost of assisted living. In some states, Medicaid may cover some of the expenses of assisted living. Generally speaking, however, assisted living costs are covered by the patient and/or their family.

Skilled nursing facilities (SNF) are health-care centers that provide 24/7 room and board, as well as care and supervision by skilled professionals. Services include nursing care, personal care, social services, and rehabilitation services. Facilities also provide medications, supplies, and other equipment. The private pay cost of an SNF ranges from about $6,000 to $9,000 per month.

There is an important distinction between a temporary SNF stay for acute illness and long-term placement for chronic care. If a person is expected to go home after stabilizing at an SNF, this is considered a temporary stay. This type of stay is covered by most insurance plans, including Medicare, as long as specific criteria are met. Long-term care placement is needed when some-one can no longer live independently due to illness or disability. Long-term care SNF placement is not covered by Medicare, nor by other insurance plans, and must either be paid for out of pocket or through a Medicaid Institutional Care Program (ICP). Medicaid is a joint federal/state program and has strict eligibility criteria based on medical and financial need. There are asset limits for the appli-cant and their spouse (if applicable), although there are assets, such as a home and a car, that are exempt. Medicaid specialists are available to assist with determining eligibility and completing the application process. Fees for this service vary.

What to Say

"Can we talk about how things are going at home for you? I'm feeling a bit worried about your well-being and want to explore some options together."

"I love you and want the best for you. I know it's really hard to think about, but I'm wondering if the safest place for you is in assisted living."

"It seems like you are needing more care now, and we cannot afford any more hours of private caregiving. I think we need to consider some other options where you can be well cared for and that we can afford."

What to Do

- Conduct a financial assessment and determine your caregiving budget.

- Track how your loved one is doing in the home setting in terms of safety.

- Track your loved one's medical needs to determine if they can be met in the home environment.

- Talk to the doctor about any concerns you have. Ask if they think you should consider long-term care placement.

- Contact the cancer care coordinator to explore options for long-term care and potential Medicaid eligibility.

- Ask friends, family, and professionals about reputable long-term care options. Visit any recommended facilities.

- Consider hiring a placement specialist. They are aware of the eligibility criteria and bed availability in local assisted living facilities.

- Slowly open the dialogue with your loved one. Approach them with empathy and compassion. Honestly share your concerns about the need to consider long-term care placement.

What to Ask a Long-Term Care Provider

1. Do you have bed availability? If not, what is the anticipated timeline for an opening?

2. What is the monthly cost?

3. What services do you provide?

4. Will my loved one be able to have a private room?

5. Is someone available to help assist us with a Medicaid application (for SNF placement)?

6. Do you have any Medicaid beds available, and if not, are you keeping a waiting list? What is the timeline?

7. What kinds of activities do you provide for residents?

8. Do you provide transportation services?

9. Do you help with ordering and administering medications?

How Are You Doing?

Coming to terms with the need for long-term care can be a stressful and emotionally draining process. Caregivers are charged with the responsibility of recognizing when more care is needed and putting an action plan into place. Securing long-term care help, whether in the home or in a facility, can be extremely time- and energy-consuming, as well as emotionally taxing. Coping with financial stress can make this all the more challenging.

Although this may be an especially difficult time for caregivers to consider their own needs, taking even 15 to 30 minutes each day for self-care can bring stress levels down. Stress, particularly chronic stress, can sometimes manifest in negative thoughts that affect both emotional and physical well-being. Incorporating a practice of affirmation-based positive thinking into your day can be an effective stress-management tool.

Affirmations are statements featuring positive, encouraging language that, if practiced over time, can begin to replace entrenched negative thought patterns. It is important that your affirmations resonate with you. Keep them brief and positive, and start them with the word "I." Read them out loud as a daily practice, and repeat as often as desired. Here are a few examples; feel free to write your own as well.

1. "I am a loving, giving person and always strive to do my best."
2. "I can manage my life with strength and resilience."
3. "I trust I am making good decisions."

4. _____

5. _____

6. _____

CHAPTER 7

Advanced Cancer Care

PETER

Eric's father, Peter, was 79 when he was diagnosed with advanced stage lymphoma, after which he underwent an aggressive chemotherapy regimen that put him into remission for two years. As the COVID-19 pandemic was breaking out, Peter began to feel unwell. With all the pandemic protocols and restrictions, it took six weeks for Peter to get medical attention. The cancer had returned "with a vengeance," and Peter was hospitalized. "My father's oncologist did not recommend chemotherapy," Eric says, "but the hospitalist encouraged my father to fight. So, we continued on with blood transfusions, but there came a point when it was clear that, unless we kept on doing transfusions, my father would quickly decline. As confusing a time as this was, I am so grateful for those extra few weeks in the hospital when we could visit. I brought him pizza, and we watched golf together." Eric noted how he and his mother "were in a battle over bringing him home or having him go to a nursing home." Ultimately, they decided to take Peter home with hospice care, and he passed away four days later: "The day he came home, I remember my mom fed him hot dogs and beans and he loved it. Then he walked to the bathroom to shave. I think he knew the end was coming. I stood next to him as he looked in the mirror, and he said to me, 'You are my hero.' Those were the last words he spoke."

Facing Advanced Cancer

The term *advanced cancer* refers to cancer that has progressed to a stage where a cure is not likely. Advanced cancer cases vary greatly from person to person and are affected by many factors, including the type of cancer and available treatment as well as a person's unique response to treatment. For some, treatment can work well, keeping the cancer at bay for years; for others, it might mean weeks to months.

For most people, receiving an advanced cancer diagnosis is a dramatic, life-altering moment. The impact can be so overwhelming initially that some may experience shock, denial, a flood of intense anxiety, or incapacitating depression. Whatever the reaction, this is a time to be as nonjudgmental and compassionate as possible. Although many of us perhaps have thought about our mortality, there is no way to truly understand what it is like to face it directly unless it is actually happening to us. Your loved one needs time to digest and integrate the reality of their situation. They also need to know they can count on their support network to honor their choices and stand by them as they navigate the many challenges ahead.

Advanced cancer treatment options vary widely. In some cases, there are several lines of treatment that can be attempted to help manage the illness. In other, less fortunate cases, the goal is to provide as much symptom relief and palliative comfort as possible. Some with treatment options may wish to do everything possible for as long as possible, whereas others may choose to forego treatment and pursue comfort care. There are also situations in which people pursue treatment for a time but choose to stop if side effects diminish their quality of life to an unsustainable point.

Facing one's own mortality calls into question one's goals and values—what's most important in a person's life and how they wish to live it. Learning to live in the midst of great uncertainty can redefine quality of life and encourage one to live fully in the present moment.

The caregiver's role becomes even more crucial during the advanced cancer stage. There may be a greater demand for both physical support and emotional caretaking, all while caregivers grapple with their own fears, sadness, and grief. Caregivers can play an instrumental role in assessing their loved one's goals of care and support them in making decisions that align with their values. Caregivers don't always agree with their loved one's choices around treatment decisions, how they care for themselves, or how they wish to spend their time. They may find it helpful to remember, with love and compassion, that this is their loved one's journey and that they must set the tone and feel empowered to make their own decisions.

What to Say

"I love you and I am here for you. It's probably going to take some time to process this."

"This is a moment in life we can't possibly prepare for. Let's take one thing at a time and look at what's right in front of us to do."

"I can only imagine how this feels. But I'm on this path with you, and I will always walk beside you and do whatever I can to support you."

"When you are up to it, it might be helpful to begin thinking about what's really important to you and how you want to spend your time."

What to Do

- Before speaking, ask your loved one if they would like to engage in conversation. It may be better to sit quietly for a bit and wait for your loved one to begin the conversation.

- Offer to assist with researching the diagnosis and treatment options.

- Begin thinking globally about what needs might arise, such as in-home caregiving, getting financial and legal matters in order, enlisting the support network, and securing emotional support for both you and your loved one.

- When it feels right, consider opening the conversation about your loved one's wishes and priorities.

- Empower your loved one to make their preferences known to their family, friends, and medical professionals.

- When appropriate, open the door to conversations about hospice care. It is easier to talk about hospice care before you actually need it.

What to Ask Your Doctor

1. What are the treatment options available?

2. Are there any clinical trials available either here or at another institution?

3. What treatment course do you recommend?

4. What are the side effects?

5. What is the anticipated life expectancy with and without treatment?

6. Are there other medical professionals, such as a palliative care team, that we can call upon to help with symptom management?

7. Can you provide referrals for support services, such as a cancer care coordinator and a dietician?

Palliative Care and Hospice

Palliative care and hospice are invaluable branches of medical care utilized for the treatment of advanced cancer. Palliative care specifically focuses on improving quality of life and providing symptom relief. A palliative care approach can be initiated at any point in the cancer care cycle and is often recommended at earlier stages to ensure that symptom management and other quality-of-life issues are addressed early.

As opposed to a broader referral spectrum for palliative care, hospice care is employed at a period called *end-of-life*. Generally speaking, a referral to hospice is initiated when a person has a prognosis (life expectancy) of six months or less. It is important to note that this does not mean the person will, in fact, die within six months, but it does mean that the seriousness of the patient's condition makes death appear to be likely in a timeline of months rather than years.

Palliative Care

Palliative care utilizes the expertise of multiple medical professionals who together, as a team, support patients and their loved ones in living the highest quality of life possible. These professionals receive specific training in palliative care and may be called palliative care specialists. The palliative care team takes a comprehensive, holistic approach to addressing the physical, mental, social, emotional, and spiritual needs of their patients. The care team composition varies but usually includes the following disciplines: medical doctors, nurses (including nurse practitioners), social workers/psychologists, and chaplains who provide spiritual support. The team may also include pharmacists and registered dieticians. Palliative care begins with an in-depth assessment that allows the providers to understand the patient's needs. Once the needs are defined, services such as medical intervention, care coordination, counseling, and advocacy can be implemented.

Some issues commonly addressed by the palliative care team include:

- Physical symptoms, such as pain, fatigue, nausea, insomnia, and loss of appetite
- Emotional issues, such as depression and anxiety
- Caregiver needs, such as dealing with burnout, coping with high stress levels, and referrals to pertinent community resources
- Legal, financial, and practical needs
- Goals of care, wishes, and priorities

Palliative care can be given in conjunction with active treatment, and palliative care team members will work closely with other members of the cancer care team. Historically speaking, palliative care has applied mostly to end-stage cancer cases, but contemporarily, it is much more widely used throughout treatment for serious and chronic diseases. In most practices, the oncologist is the ideal first person to ask for information about palliative care and how to obtain a referral. Palliative care is typically covered by private health insurance and may be covered, at least in part, by Medicare and Medicaid.

Hospice

Hospice services provide holistic care to improve quality of life for patients and their loved ones, typically in the end-of-life stage. Hospice services are overseen by a medical doctor who serves as the hospice medical director. Direct care is provided by an interdisciplinary team often consisting of a nurse case manager, a social worker, a home health aide, a chaplain, and trained volunteers. Each hospice team member has a specific role; however, it is up to patients and their families to decide which services they would like to utilize. In the event of a crisis or after-hours need, there is generally an on-call nurse available 24/7 to answer calls and make a hospice home visit.

Hospice services can be provided in a variety of locations:

- Home hospice care is delivered in the patient's home. The hospice team members make regular visits at specific, determined intervals. Because home hospice care is not 24-hour care, a primary caregiver must be named and willing to oversee the caregiving needs.
- Hospital-based hospices are offered in the hospital setting.
- Inpatient hospice facilities provide 24/7 care.
- Long-term care facilities may have hospice units or work closely with hospices in the community that come in to provide care.

Although the treating physician often initiates the conversation about hospice care, anyone can contact hospices and request an informational visit. Hospice services are covered by Medicare and the Department of Veterans Affairs (VA) and may also be covered by Medicaid, depending on the state. For those with private insurance, coverage varies, so it is best to contact your insurance provider for specific details. For those who are uninsured or whose plan doesn't fully cover services, many hospices may offer care for free or at a reduced cost thanks to fundraising efforts and donations.

What to Say

"I want you to have the best quality of life possible. It sounds like that's the focus of the palliative care team. I can follow up and make an appointment when and if you'd like to see them."

"I think it might be a good idea to meet with the palliative care team. The doctor said they could help with managing symptoms, and I imagine that could be really helpful."

"There are a lot of misconceptions about hospice care and the best time for it. Hospice care offers so many important services, and I think hospice help could make a major difference for us sooner rather than later."

What to Do

- Talk with your loved one about what they feel they need. Make a list of their issues and concerns. This can be a springboard for a conversation about enlisting palliative care or hospice services.

- If you have private insurance, see if palliative care and hospice services are covered and to what extent.

- Encourage your loved one to take advantage of services that are offered. It might be helpful to tell them how valuable the services are for caregivers as well as patients.

- If hospice care is appropriate for your loved one and you have options when it comes to providers, interview multiple hospices.

- Assess the caregiving situation at home. If hospice care is appropriate, determine whether it's best for your loved one to receive care in the home, in an inpatient facility, or in a nursing home that provides hospice services.

What to Ask Your Doctor

1. Do you think a referral for a palliative care consult is appropriate at this point?

2. What signs would indicate a hospice referral is appropriate?

3. If we sign on with hospice, can we still connect with you? Will you still be overseeing the care? How does that work?

4. Is there a specific hospice you would recommend? Should we speak to the cancer care team about connecting with some options?

5. Do you recommend home hospice care, or do you think our needs would be better met in an inpatient hospice?

End-of-Life Decisions

When a loved one enters the end-of-life phase, many questions, concerns, and emotions may arise. When there are no more treatment options and anticipated life expectancy is limited, optimizing quality of life and minimizing suffering become the highest priorities. Some families have already had conversations about their loved one's wishes and have legal documents in order. Others may not have had the time or opportunity and may now have to scramble for arrangements, making this period even more challenging.

The first step in assisting a loved one during this time is determining what their wishes are regarding their medical care. At this juncture, some people may not want any medical intervention and may solely want to be kept as comfortable as possible. One way to prevent unwanted medical intervention is to execute a *Do Not Resuscitate (DNR)* order. The patient's physician signs this form, which explicitly refuses CPR (cardiopulmonary resuscitation) if the patient's heart or breathing stops. This document is posted in the home in an easy-to-see place. In the event that someone calls 911, the paramedics will see the DNR, know your loved one's wishes, and not intervene with CPR. As discussed earlier, it is also very helpful to execute a living will and Durable Power of Attorney for Health Care.

Another important question is whether someone wishes to pass at home or in the hospital. For those that wish to pass at home (whether in their personal home or a nursing home), hospice is one of the most valuable resources. With quality of life as their explicit goal, the hospice team brings expertise in comfort care and symptom management. Home health aides provide personal care, and social workers can assist with a multitude of practical matters and provide counseling and emotional support. Hospice chaplains provide spiritual support, and volunteers can run errands, provide respite, and help with household tasks for which caregivers may not have the time or energy. When there is a crisis, instead of calling 911, families are instructed to call hospice. A hospice nurse is available by phone and through in-person visits to help families work through challenges in the home setting. They provide education so caregivers can become more comfortable administering medications and doing other critical tasks. Some people have the preconceived notion that hospice is only appropriate weeks or days before someone passes. However, the earlier hospice help is enlisted, the greater the benefits for both patients and families.

Caregivers may also face the difficult question of whether there are enough personal and financial resources to keep their loved one at home. Someone at end-of-life requires around-the-clock care, even with hospice involvement. Although the support network may be able to cover the caregiving needs, sometimes a nursing home placement needs to be considered.

One of the more challenging topics to broach is that of funeral arrangements. However, asking your loved one directly about their wishes reduces stress and confusion in the long run. It also brings comfort and peace of mind knowing you are properly carrying out their wishes. Ask important questions like whether they want to be buried or cremated, what type of service they may want (if any), and if they want to be an organ donor. If hospice is involved, they can help facilitate this conversation and provide resource information.

End-of-life decision-making is challenging under the best of circumstances, but it is even more difficult when family members have disagreements. Your loved one's wishes and values should be the compass that guides decision-making, not the potentially differing opinions of family members or friends.

Sometimes, it is not possible to know your loved one's wishes. They may be physically and/or cognitively impaired or find the topic upsetting. Under such circumstances, caregivers will make decisions based on what they believe is in the best interests of their loved one. If there is family strife, hospice personnel can facilitate family meetings, or a private therapist can be hired to assist.

What to Say

"We are at a point where some important decisions need to be made. I would like to know your wishes and priorities."

"Sometimes people get to a point where they don't want any more medical intervention. Can we talk about what kind of medical care you may or may not want at this point in time?"

"I know these topics might be hard to talk about. They are for me, too, but knowing what is important to you is my highest priority, even if it's hard to talk about."

"When you are up to it, I would like to talk about options for getting help at home."

What to Do

- Assess the caregiving situation. Anticipating your loved one's decline, think through options for increased caregiving in the home, such as enlisting your support network and/or hiring help.

- Ask your loved one if they are open to a hospice informational visit.

- If there are legal documents expressing your loved one's wishes, find them and read them over carefully with your loved one, if able. Ascertain whether any updates are needed.

- If a nursing home placement is needed at any point and hospice is involved, they can help facilitate the transfer. If hospice is not involved, consider reaching out to the cancer care coordinator through the oncology program and seeing what resources and information they can offer. You can also contact nursing homes directly.

- If you are unclear about your loved one's wishes, open the discussion gently and address one issue at a time.

What to Ask Your Doctor

1. At what point do you recommend executing a Do Not Resuscitate (DNR) order?

2. Is a referral to hospice appropriate at this time? What signs should we be looking for to help us determine when more care is needed?

3. What can we expect as time goes by, in terms of how the body will change and decline?

4. How can we best prepare for the changes that are coming?

5. How will we know that death may be near? What are some of the signs we should watch for?

How Are You Doing?

As a caregiver for someone moving through the end-of-life phase, it may be difficult to put any attention on yourself. People may ask you if there's anything they can do, and you may not be able to answer them because you haven't had any time or energy to consider the question. Caregivers are consumed with ensuring that their loved one has the care they need and that they are made as comfortable as possible. Many provide 24/7 care with minimal respite. In addition to the physical demands of caregiving, there are many other important arenas that require a caregiver's attention and care. It may be a challenge to eat properly or stay adequately hydrated, and your sleep may be disrupted. A caregiver's emotional needs may also be put on the back burner. There may not be time to see friends, attend a support group, or connect with a therapist for emotional support.

The following is a simple relaxation exercise that can help relieve stress, even during this most demanding caregiving phase.

1. Sit in a comfortable chair or lie down.
2. Take a couple deep breaths.
3. Starting at your feet, tense the muscles in them for 5 to 10 seconds, then release. Notice the relaxation you feel in your feet.
4. Work your way up your body, tensing and releasing each muscle group—feet, legs, pelvis, abdomen, chest, arms, hands, shoulders, and face.
5. Notice your body's response to this relaxing exercise. Sit for another moment to enjoy the feelings of relaxation.

PART 3

Caring for Yourself

A caregiver's journey can be a rugged one, profoundly affecting your physical, mental, and emotional well-being. Many caregivers are stretched to their limits, with self-care often falling by the wayside. Caregivers may be so consumed with assisting their loved one that they may not have any idea how the demands of the caregiving role are affecting them or know how to balance their lives. These next chapters will identify how the caregiving role impacts health and offer practical tools for finding support and integrating self-care into your daily life.

CHAPTER 8

How Caregiving Affects You

NOAH

Noah and Dalia were busy raising their three children when Noah was diagnosed with stage IV lung cancer at age 40. Noah was given a prognosis of months to a few years, but he has endured 15 years of the disease and treatments. As a long-term caregiver, Dalia looks back on the many challenges she has faced: "I became Mom and Dad to the children, all while needing to care for Noah, too. I did my best." Dalia recalls they didn't always agree about how to manage the cancer. "Guilt has been the hardest thing for me. There were times when I wanted him to do everything to fight. But I have learned that this is his disease, not mine, and ultimately he needs to make the decisions."

Dalia attributes her resilience to many factors, including her own challenging childhood, which "allowed me to develop into a leader early on and helped me quickly take charge after the diagnosis and recognize what needed to be done." She also recalls the benefits of a support group, her therapy sessions, and their vast support network.

In recent years, Noah's disease has spread to his brain and compromised his cognitive abilities. "We can't talk the way we used to, and I am grieving the loss of my partner. Sometimes I want to run away or I just feel so done." But Dalia's strength prevails. "With all that we have faced, everything becomes more immediate. I can only think in terms of days to a month. This has taught me to live in the moment."

The Emotional and Physical Toll

The role of the caregiver can be extremely demanding, rippling through all areas of life. Caregivers are called into action from the moment a loved one is diagnosed. They must not only tend to an onslaught of practical matters but also be available to emotionally support their loved one as they face one of the greatest challenges of their lives.

No matter how demanding or prolonged the caregiving situation is, a caregiver's experience is both physically and emotionally taxing. One of the more common symptoms caregivers contend with is fatigue. From attending appointments to researching treatments, from coordinating care to keeping the household running, caregivers are consistently in a mode of doing. Over time, the exhaustion can accumulate, especially if a caregiver is, for whatever reason, not able to practice reliable and sufficient self-care.

Caregiving can affect the quality and quantity of sleep, which can contribute to fatigue and compromise physical and mental health. Worry, fear, sadness, or grief can make it difficult to fall or stay asleep. It is important to address sleep issues as early as possible. There are a variety of approaches that can help, including pharmaceutical interventions and mind-body stress management practices.

Feelings of sadness and depression are also common among caregivers. Watching a loved one contend with the challenges of cancer can feel heartbreaking, and cancer can bring many losses. Your relationship with your loved one may have dramatically changed, and you may not be able to engage with each other as you once could. Other strong emotions such as guilt, fear, and anger may also arise, and a general feeling of anxiety can pervade daily life.

These stresses and strains can lead to *caregiver burnout*. Caregiver burnout is a state in which the physical, mental, and emotional burdens of caregiving have reached a maximum level and the caregiver's health and well-being are in jeopardy.

Sometimes burnout can set in because caregivers don't have respite care and cannot get breaks, perhaps due to a lack of financial resources or a limited support network. Some caregivers have access to resources but feel guilty using them, putting an undue burden on themselves to manage everything on their own. Long-term, chronic emotional stress can also contribute to burnout. Signs of caregiver burnout are similar to signs of depression: withdrawal from loved ones, a persistent sad or irritable mood, feelings of hopelessness, changes in sleeping and eating patterns, and loss of interest in activities that once brought pleasure.

Remember that you are not alone on this path. It is normal and appropriate to experience symptoms of caregiver stress, to feel fatigued and experience emotional ups and downs. Caregivers are taxed in unimaginable ways. Tending to a loved one's physical and emotional needs while problem-solving and managing practical matters is a full-time job. Finding time for self-care may be difficult and may consistently be pushed aside because the demands of the caregiving role feel more pressing and important.

Like most things in life, recognizing issues before they become problems is ideal. The sooner a caregiver recognizes that self-care is vital, the better they will function. It is important to build a support network early on and to learn ways to manage stress. Obtaining professional counseling, attending a support group, and spending quality time with family and friends can reduce stress considerably. Other self-care practices such as exercise, good nutrition, adequate rest, and daily relaxation time can all help reduce the emotional and physical toll of caregiving.

Stress and Anxiety

Stress and anxiety are part of the human experience. Life can present many challenges, and early on we learn ways to cope with our difficulties. If we are fortunate, we are able to manage the stress associated with loss, disappointment, change, and transition. But there are times when life can become more difficult to manage.

Although a certain level of anxiety is likely to be manageable, there are some signs and symptoms that may require attention and support:

- Feeling keyed up, nervous, or physically tense
- Rapid heart rate
- Feeling shaky or trembling
- Overheating or sweating excessively
- Difficulty concentrating
- Excessive worrying
- Feelings of dread or panic
- Difficulty falling or staying asleep and/or restless sleep

If you are experiencing such symptoms, remember that you are in one of life's most stressful situations. Be kind to yourself. These warning signs are friendly reminders that your stress levels may be at a critical point. Rule out any medical causes by reporting symptoms to your doctor.

Frustration and Anger

Though anger and frustration are common reactions, when they arise it may feel like there is no place for them under the circumstances. A caregiver may ask, "How can I possibly feel anger or frustration when my loved one is dealing with cancer?" It is important that these feelings be acknowledged and honored. It is okay to be angry that your loved one got cancer and that your lives have changed dramatically as a result. It is understandable that being overwhelmed with responsibility may make you feel irritable and frustrated. It's also possible that some things your loved one says or does may trigger such feelings. This is all part of the coping process.

If you find it difficult to contain your emotions, begin to lash out in anger, or find yourself in more disagreements with your loved ones, it is important to acknowledge those feelings and reach out to family and friends for support or obtain professional help.

Sadness and Depression

All who are touched by cancer are very likely to experience sadness and depression. Although these are common and very understandable emotions, there are times when they may be cause for concern. If you are plagued by persistent sadness, you may be suffering from depression. Some signs and symptoms include:

- Changes in appetite resulting in weight gain or loss
- Changes in sleep patterns, such as sleeping too much or too little
- Increased irritability
- Persistent sad or depressed mood
- Feelings of helplessness/hopelessness
- Excessive tiredness
- Frequent crying episodes
- Loss of pleasure in activities you once enjoyed
- Low self-esteem or being hard on yourself
- Thoughts of self-harm

Some caregivers may already have a history of depression and may have sought professional help or tried medication. Others may be experiencing depression for the first time, which can feel frightening and overwhelming. There are various levels of depression, from low-grade to severe, and the interventions needed will vary. Wherever you may fall on the continuum, it is important to talk to someone about how you are feeling. If the depression is interfering with your functioning, impacting your relationships, or prohibiting you from participating in life, strongly consider seeking professional help.

Guilt

One of the more painful feelings caregivers grapple with is guilt, constantly asking themselves if they could be doing more.

Experiencing guilt is common for those on the caregiving journey. You want the best for your loved one and may have unreasonably high expectations of yourself in the caregiving role. The reality is that the job of the caregiver is immense, and it may be very difficult or impossible to meet every single need that arises.

Coping with guilt is not easy, but here are some ways to better manage it:

- Acknowledge the feelings as a normal part of the caregiving experience.
- Reach out to a trusted person to talk about it.
- Ease up on yourself and hold yourself with compassion.
- Rethink your expectations to make them more manageable.

Exhaustion and Physical Issues

Although it may feel rewarding to serve as a caregiver, it can require an immense output of physical and emotional energy. Even the most resilient caregiver will suffer from exhaustion, especially if the caregiving spans a lengthy period. Caregivers may learn to live with fatigue and other physical symptoms, unaware of the detrimental effects of their self-neglect. If a caregiver suffers from burnout, it could compromise the quality of the care they provide and endanger their own health and well-being.

Physical signs of caregiver burnout include:

- Debilitating fatigue
- Decreased ability to cope with daily stress
- Physical changes, such as weight gain or loss
- Sleep problems
- Immune issues, such as frequent colds or flu
- Pain
- Digestive issues
- Headaches
- Social isolation or withdrawal from friends and family
- Increased use of drugs or alcohol

What to Do

- Check in with yourself honestly. Focus on symptoms of stress overload, depression, and caregiver burnout.

- Prioritize what you need to do in your day. Let the simple steps be enough.

- Reach out to a trusted friend or family member to talk about how you are feeling.

- Consider speaking with your doctor about how to manage stress and whether pharmaceutical intervention is needed.

- If you don't already have a therapist and have the means, consider getting one.

- If inclined, join a caregiver support group. Your cancer care coordinator can provide information on options in your area.

- Think about ways your support network can help reduce stress. Consider delegating some tasks.

- Take note of your eating habits and sleep quality. Are your basic needs being met?

- Be kind to yourself. Plan a nurturing activity, such as taking a warm bath or going on a walk in nature.

What to Ask Your Doctor

1. Being a caregiver is very stressful. Do you have any recommendations for how to manage the stress?

2. What can I do to get better, more restful sleep?

3. Do you know of any resources that can help with caregiver stress?

4. What signs and symptoms indicate the need for medication?

5. How can I support my immune system while enduring such stressful times?

6. Can you provide a referral for someone I can talk to, such as a social worker or therapist?

Grief and Loss

Anyone whose life has been touched by cancer will likely experience the painful feelings associated with grief and loss. *Grief* refers to feelings that arise when someone experiences a loss. A *loss* is something or someone that was once available but now is not. Grief is a natural response to loss.

From the time of diagnosis, when the doctor utters the words "You have cancer," cancer survivors must contend with the loss of health. From there, the losses can accumulate. Similarly, caregivers' lives are altered at the moment of diagnosis. Caregivers may experience a loss of innocence as they recognize their loved one is vulnerable and could be lost to the disease. Dreams and plans may need to be put on hold or released altogether. The relationship may need to shift and change in reaction to the demands of treatment, and caregivers may feel like their loved one isn't the person they once were.

Grief can be both a transient physical and emotional experience, manifesting as pain, increased blood pressure and heart rate, restlessness, physical exhaustion, nausea and vomiting, and digestive problems. Strong emotions such as fear, worry, anger, frustration, irritability, and sadness may arise.

Grief is not a linear process. Although there are various stages of grief, they are not experienced in a specific order until a conclusion is reached. Instead, people may go in and out of the various stages, in no particular order, and may revisit stages multiple times.

Several models have been developed to describe the grieving process. One of the more well-known is the five stages of grief from Elisabeth Kübler-Ross, which are denial, anger, bargaining, depression, and acceptance. Caregivers may begin grieving as early as the time of diagnosis, or they may begin to process their grief at some point during the illness. If a loved one passes, the grieving process may not begin until after the death or well into the bereavement period. Understand that everyone processes grief in their own way. There is no "right" way to grieve, nor is there a timeline for when a grieving process should be completed.

Sometimes a person's journey with cancer is so full of pain and suffering that caregivers may feel a sense of relief when a loved one has passed away. This is a common and understandable response. As sad as they may feel about losing their loved one, knowing they are no longer suffering or in pain is a comfort. Some caregivers may feel guilty for their feelings of relief. It is important to let yourself feel the feelings so they can move through you and ultimately dissipate.

Losing a precious loved one or watching them suffer can leave a person feeling inconsolable. Sometimes nothing can be said or done to make them feel better. Rather, it is a process that people must move through in their own way and time. Let the feelings arise and find outlets for expression, whether with friends and family, a support group, individual counseling, or spiritual counseling.

Self-care is of paramount importance during the grieving process. Attending to physical needs can help keep a person strong as they tend to their emotional needs. Meditation, yoga, visualization, and breathing exercises can help relieve stress and create more space to process feelings. Creative outlets such as painting, writing, or playing a musical instrument can be vehicles for self-expression.

Be careful not to compare yourself to others as you move through the grieving process. Seek out support in whatever form resonates with you. Remember that you are in the midst of one of life's most difficult chapters. As always, hold yourself with kindness and compassion.

What to Do

- Take time to rest. Processing grief takes energy.

- Consider taking time off from work if you are able to do so.

- When emotions come up, allow yourself to feel them.

- Reach out to your support network for emotional support and/or practical help.

- Be kind and gentle with yourself.

- Release expectations about how you might feel. The bereavement process is different for everyone.

- Take care of your body with good nutrition and exercise.

- Get outside every day if possible.

- Attend a support group, if you are so inclined. Many hospices offer bereavement support groups to the general public that are free or low cost.

- Connect with emotional and/or spiritual support. Consider bereavement counseling, therapy, or connecting with your religious leader, if applicable.

What to Ask Your Therapist, Religious Leader, or Trusted Friends

1. I feel so guilty, like I could have done more. What can I do to deal with these feelings?

2. I feel like I'm in shock, as if my loved one is going to walk through the door any minute. Is that normal?

3. I'm having trouble sleeping. Do you have any ideas as to what might help me?

4. I feel lonely. Do you know of any groups or resources that could help?

5. I'm feeling some anger coming up. Is that expected?

6. I'm thinking about what happens when people die. What do you think happens?

7. Are there spiritual practices that can help ease my grief?

How Are You Doing?

A caregiver is at their best when they can find the balance between meeting the needs of their loved one and caring for themselves. If you have taken the time to read this book, you have already taken a great step forward by recognizing the complicated nature of the caregiving role. Keeping a journal may provide added balance.

Journaling can be an outlet for expressing your feelings and identifying your needs, and it can serve as a vehicle for self-exploration and problem-solving.

Journaling can be simple. You can journal as long and as often as you like, with pen and paper or on your computer. To start, try setting aside 10 minutes in a quiet place, and consider the following questions:

1. How am I feeling?
2. What do I need?
3. What can I do to take care of myself today?

CHAPTER 9

Work-Life Balance

AVA

Lina's sister, Ava, was diagnosed with breast cancer at age 46. Ava's husband traveled often for work, and Lina stepped in as primary caregiver. "I feel so blessed I got to be a part of her care and to be with her when she needed me," Lina says.

Lina worked full-time while caregiving and learned how to balance her responsibilities. She was able to work remotely, which made it possible to continue working while functioning as a caregiver. Lina felt "lucky [to have] a great boss who was understanding and coworkers who were supportive."

When it was necessary to take time off, Lina used personal days or sick days and requested a leave of absence when her sister needed more care. "Thankfully, I could divide my time between work and caregiving," she explains. "We also had help from other family members, which filled in the gaps." Through out her caregiving experiences, Lina was able to use massage, acupressure, and therapy to help keep her strong and resilient. She credits humor as one of her greatest coping strategies: "We giggled together and joked with each other, but we could also talk about the illness. Tragedies bring you closer. My experiences helped me see life as something you can't change but you do the best you can to get through."

Balancing Work and Caregiving

For many caregivers, work is an essential component of their lives. With only so many hours in a day, caregivers are forced to balance their work and their caregiving role. A caregiver's ability to take time off or obtain a flexible schedule varies greatly. Some caregivers may be self-employed and have no benefits, and time off must be taken without pay. Others may work for companies that offer flexible hours and benefits such as health insurance, sick leave, paid time off, and job protection through the Family and Medical Leave Act (FMLA).

When a loved one is diagnosed, working caregivers must determine their employer's policies and procedures regarding caregiving, including employees' legal rights. This is best accomplished by contacting the company's human resources department or company administrator to discuss the following points:

- The availability of paid time off (PTO), sick days, or vacation days that may be used for caregiving
- Policies regarding a leave of absence and the Family and Medical Leave Act (FMLA)
- Strategies for talking with management about the need for time off

The Family and Medical Leave Act is a 1993 federal law that allows eligible employees to take up to 12 weeks of unpaid leave and provides both job protection and continued health-care coverage during time off. FMLA coverage applies to private sector employers who have 50 or more employees and all public agencies, including schools. Employers with less than 50 employees are not covered by FMLA; however, protection may be granted at the state level. FMLA covers those who have been employed for at least 12 months and have worked at least 1,250 hours within the last year. Human resources representatives are well versed in company leave policies and are the best source of information for employees on their rights.

When speaking with management, it is important to be as transparent as possible about the situation. It may be difficult to know what your needs are going to be, so let your manager know that there are some unknowns. Be honest about how the demands of the caregiving situation may affect work. Determine whether a flexible schedule is possible, allowing for time off to accompany your loved one to appointments and for other necessary caregiving tasks. Also consider inquiring whether working remotely will be acceptable when needed. For those who can manage financially on a reduced income, there may be the option of job sharing or reducing hours to a part-time status. Many employers are open to working with their employees to meet the needs of all involved.

How much personal information employees disclose to their managers depends on the situation. Those with supportive managers may choose to share more openly about their home responsibilities. This will help managers understand what your needs are and how they can support you during these stressful times. However, employees are *not* required to divulge the details of their loved one's circumstances to their managers. You need only to state that you need time off to take care of a family member.

What to Do

- Know your rights. Contact your company's HR department to find out what you are entitled to as a caregiver regarding paid time off, unpaid leave, and qualifying for FMLA.

- As best you can, determine your need for time off. Come to your manager with a plan for balancing work with your caregiving responsibilities, whether that means working a flexible schedule, working remotely, or cutting back hours if needed.

- Be clear that there are many unknowns when it comes to cancer, should you choose to discuss the specifics of the illness with your employer. Discuss a contingency plan for urgent situations.

- If you work in a supportive environment, let your manager and coworkers know more details about your caregiving situation and how they can help lighten your load.

What to Ask Your Manager or HR Department

1. I will need to take time off to care for my loved one. Do I have any paid time off available? If so, how much? What do I need to do to request time off?

2. Is the company covered under FMLA? Am I entitled to 12 weeks of unpaid leave with job protection and continuation of health coverage?

3. Can I possibly work a flexible schedule so I can be available for any daytime appointments?

4. Is it possible to reduce my hours and go to part-time status? How would this affect my income and benefits?

Asking for Help

One of the most essential qualities of a resilient caregiver is the ability to ask for help. For some, this can be very uncomfortable, and they may choose to avoid it. Sometimes caregivers have unrealistic expectations of themselves and try to take on more than one person can handle. For such caregivers, it's only a matter of time before burnout sets in.

Caregiving is not meant to be a solitary job; it's a shared responsibility. Family members, friends, coworkers, and other community members are likely poised and ready to help if called upon. They often feel helpless and need direction as to what they can do. Vague offers of help are usually born out of a lack of awareness and understanding of what is truly needed. It is important to take inventory and determine ways your support network can help.

Sometimes caregivers are so overwhelmed it may be difficult to take time to assess their needs, but in the long run it is time well spent. It is important to look inward and be honest about how much you can do on your own and what can be realistically delegated.

It is ideal to mobilize your support network early. The first step is identifying who is included. Consider family, friends, neighbors, coworkers, and community members. There are also online resources, such as forums where caregivers can offer emotional support and share resources. As discussed in chapter 6 (page 93), sometimes hiring help is necessary if within your budget.

After identifying who is in your support network, determine what kind of help is needed. Mentally retrace how your days are spent, and think through what needs to be accomplished. Make a list of what you must do and what can be delegated. Consider breaking down the needs into categories such as meals, transportation, errands, home maintenance and housekeeping, doctor's appointments, pet care and/or childcare, respite care, personal care for your loved one, and medication management.

Now that you have identified who is in your support network and what is needed, reach out and ask for help. One strategy to consider is having a point person, such as a trusted friend or family member, channel requests for help to the support network. This can take the pressure off the caregiver having to directly ask for help from myriad sources. Stay in close touch with your point person, giving them honest direction and detailed specifics about what is needed.

There are also websites dedicated to supporting caregivers. These sites offer communication tools you can use to ask for help and keep your support network updated. Some include a calendar feature that can be used to sign up for specific tasks such as preparing meals, running errands, and accompanying your loved one to their appointments. Several websites also have free, downloadable, user-friendly apps that can streamline the caregiving process. More information is provided in the Resources section on page 158.

Caregiving is a long-term process and requires sustained energy. The more you let yourself reach out for help, the better you will be able to care for yourself and your loved one during this time.

What to Do

- Ask yourself how everyday life could be easier if you had a bit more help and support. Remember those who care about you and who have expressed a desire to help. They simply need some direction from you.

- Make a list of your support network. Be sure to include coworkers, neighbors, and community members.

- Make a list of tasks that can be delegated to your support network. Think about who in the support network might be best equipped for each task.

- Consider talking with a friend or family member who can manage the support network in terms of communication and coordinating help.

- Hold regularly scheduled family meetings for updates and care planning.

What to Ask Your Family and Friends

1. We could use some help with transportation to appointments on days that I am working. Would you be available to help out, and if so, what might your schedule permit?

2. I need to get some documents in order and make some difficult decisions. It would be helpful if you could assist me with this. Are you available, and if so, when?

3. I really need to get out and take a break. Would you be able to come watch over things while I'm gone?

4. Could you possibly be our point person and handle coordinating help for us?

Outside Services

There are a vast variety of resources available that can help you save time, energy, and potentially money. Although some national programs provide services locally, there are also local programs that vary widely from community to community. A good place to begin is the American Cancer Society, which you can call at 1-800-ACS-2345. A representative will search their database for available services near you.

Meal preparation. Some home-delivery meal companies offer fully prepared meals, while others offer meal kits with recipes and ingredients that can typically be prepared in 30 minutes or less. Costs can be as low as $2.49 per serving. Read the reviews to help discern which program is best for your needs.

Community agencies may also provide free or low-cost meals to cancer survivors and their families. Look online or call the American Cancer Society for information about your specific community's offerings.

Grocery delivery. Having your groceries or other household necessities delivered saves time and energy. Again, there are many choices, including organic food delivery services. Search online for options in your area.

Laundry services. Whatever you may pay in dollars for laundry services will be returned to you in time. There are a variety of laundry services (wash, dry, and fold) available that vary in cost.

Housekeeping. There are organizations that provide free or low-cost housekeeping services to cancer survivors. One organization that provides services to cancer patients in all 50 states and Canada is Cleaning for a Reason.

If you have hired caregiving help, consider asking for assistance with housekeeping and other chores. You can also hire housekeepers through an agency (always check reviews) or private hire. If you privately hire housekeepers, get recommendations from trusted people.

Transportation. The American Cancer Society has a volunteer transportation program called Road to Recovery that provides free rides for cancer patients to and from medical appointments. For more information about registering for this program in your area, call the American Cancer Society.

Check online for other programs that provide financial assistance for transportation. Your cancer care coordinator is also a good resource for connecting with available services.

Yard care. A professional can take care of your lawn and other landscaping needs. Ask neighbors and friends for referrals, or look online and check reviews for companies in your area.

What to Do

- Contact your cancer care coordinator and ask what outside services are available.

- Think about ways to simplify your life. Make a list of the tasks that take the most time.

- For each item you wish to farm out, search online for available resources.

- Call the American Cancer Society (1-800-ACS-2345) and tell them what type of help you are looking for so they can search their database and connect you with resources and services.

- If finances are a concern, apply for programs that provide free or low-cost services, such as Cleaning for a Reason.

- Save time by having your groceries delivered or using a home-delivery meal program.

- Consider shopping online. Most stores offer this option.

What to Ask Prospective Service Providers

1. Please tell me about any packages you offer that may help with cost savings.

2. How much advance notice do you need to set up rides?

3. Do you offer any discounts for people who are going through cancer treatment?

4. For your meal delivery services, do you work on a subscription basis?

5. Are there any hidden fees to be aware of, such as delivery charges?

6. Does your program provide cash assistance, such as money for gas?

7. What types of cleaning services do you provide?

How Are You Doing?

Caregiving is a balancing act on all levels. Caregivers must learn to tend to the demands of their role while nurturing their own well-being. That said, caregivers who utilize their support network and take advantage of the wide range of resources available are much more likely to maintain resilience. Practicing self-care is equally important. Although caregivers may not have the time or the resources to get relaxing and time-consuming spa treatments or indulgences, some gentle techniques done at home can help release tension and discomfort.

- Sit or lie down in a comfortable, quiet place. Take a few moments to tune into your body. Notice where you are holding tension or where there is discomfort.

- Gently place your hands on the affected area. This simple act can be therapeutic and begin to bring healing to the area. Bring awareness to your breathing.
- You may want to gently rub the area using your fingertips in little circular motions. You can also gently squeeze the area with one hand, applying light pressure.
- Areas such as the head or scalp, face, shoulders, arms, abdomen, lower back, legs, and feet can hold a lot of tension and might be good places to focus on as you explore this simple method of self-care.

CHAPTER 10

Staying Healthy and Resilient

NIA

At 59, Judy's wife, Nia, was diagnosed with a rare type of multiple myeloma. They both had busy, full lives with demanding careers, yet Judy recalls feeling like she could no longer see the future: "You realize the life you envisioned together and have been talking about for the last 29 years has all changed." As the demands of Nia's treatment increased, Judy quietly began to take on more responsibilities, such as the cooking, cleaning, and yard work, but kept her own life going as well. "Nia didn't want me to stop my life or to let her life consume mine," she says. Judy was committed to her self-care regimen, which included seeing an acupuncturist regularly, attending tai chi classes, and making weekly dates with friends. Having spent years in therapy, Judy was aware of the relationship dynamics and the triggers that would lead to tension. "I made a decision to do my best to keep my emotions in check. Nothing was worth arguing over. We were able to talk about everything. We came together as a team, and our love intensified."

After Nia passed away, Judy attended an LGBTQ partner loss support group for three years. "I was never someone that was drawn to group activities, but it was definitely the best decision I made. I learned so much from the group about life and how to cope with loss. I also began working with a spiritual teacher and have continued to this day. It's important to find something that helps you connect and that soothes your heart."

Get Moving

Staying active can benefit your physical and mental health, and it's even more essential when caregiving. Moving the body regularly helps boost energy and immune function, combat fatigue, improve sleep, and regulate mood. Physical activity also invites social contact, which can make it more stimulating and fun if a caregiver primarily spends time with their loved one and could benefit from seeing other people.

If you are struggling to get moving, it may be helpful to expand your concept of "physical activity." It can be as simple as a gentle morning stretch or as intensive as a marathon. The key is coming up with a movement routine that is right for you in duration, frequency, and type of activity. Here are a few types of movement to consider:

- Walking can be done anywhere. You can slowly increase your pace and distance over time. Walking can give you access to nature, which for many can bring interconnected feelings of peace, serenity, and happiness.
- Stretching and yoga help promote flexibility and balance and build strength. They can be done at home or in an in-person class. There are also a multitude of online tutorials and classes that provide accessibility and convenience.
- Jogging, running, and cycling can provide a higher-intensity aerobic workout outdoors.
- Gym memberships offer a wide variety of fitness options, including exercise machines for cardio and strength training and group exercise classes.
- If you have access to a pool, try swimming, which incorporates both cardio and strength training.
- Dancing builds strength and stamina and is fun and enlivening.
- Tai chi and qigong are movement practices that help build strength, flexibility, and balance.

What to Do

- Incorporate movement into everyday life. Park the car further from the store. Take the stairs whenever possible. If you are working, walk during your lunchtime and breaks.

- Plan physical activities with your loved one when their energy permits. Consider a daily walk, if possible. Walks can be any distance, ranging from going down the block to longer hikes in nature.

- Take a movement class together, such as yoga, qigong, strength training, or cardio. Talk about what you are both interested in, and pick a class that works for both of you.

- Mark your physical activity down in your calendar, prioritizing it as an important appointment.

- Save time by incorporating social connection into your physical activities. Walk or hike with friends and family, or invite someone to join you at the gym.

What to Ask Your Doctor

1. Are there any physical activities I should avoid?

2. Are there any types of exercise you recommend more than others for someone with my health background?

3. Are there any tests or workups needed before I can start my exercise regimen?

4. Could any of my medications possibly interfere with my exercise tolerance?

Eat Right

Caregivers need sustained energy and a balanced mood in order to maintain resilience. Poor nutrition can contribute to caregiver burnout.

It is important that caregivers eat consistently and avoid going more than four to five hours without eating. Skipping meals can lead to blood sugar imbalance and cause a host of problems, including weakness, fatigue, and irritability. It is also important to stay hydrated. Many people suffer from chronic dehydration and aren't even aware of it. Some signs include fatigue, dry mouth, and light-headedness. You can make hydration more palatable by making "spa" water in the morning: Add fruit (such as lemon, lime, or orange slices), cucumbers, basil, or mint to your water.

One simple way to help maintain good nutrition is to make nutritious food easily accessible. Foods that have a combination of protein, carbohydrates, and fats are good options. Stock the pantry with nuts, nut butters, and seeds, and consider combining them with a piece of whole-grain bread or whole-grain crackers, perhaps with fruit. Keep sources of protein on hand, such as canned tuna, sardines, and canned beans. Protein smoothies are easy to digest, nutritious, and they taste good, too! Whole food sources of protein such as organic silken tofu are ideal for smoothies, but if you want to use a protein powder, look for a simple, pure one with a minimum number of ingredients. As a general guideline, do your best to minimize sugars and highly processed foods.

Consider batch cooking or meal prep when possible, preparing several portions of meals at one time to avoid having to cook on a daily basis. Keep your refrigerator and freezer stocked with easy meals. Consider getting a good cookbook, such as *The Cancer Diet Cookbook* by Dionne Detraz, which provides 30-minute, 5-ingredient, and one-pot meal recipes that both you and your loved one can enjoy.

If your budget allows, consider utilizing one of the many healthy meal delivery services available, such as Sunbasket and

Green Chef, or grocery delivery from companies such as Amazon Fresh and Instacart. Some local grocery store chains offer their own delivery services as well.

What to Do

- Eat regularly. Avoid skipping meals.
- Make eating healthy nonnegotiable and prioritize it as much as you do your loved one's nutritional needs.
- Keep easy snacks available, such as low-sugar trail mix and crackers with nut butter.
- Combine fruit with nuts instead of eating fruit alone.
- Make water easily available so you can stay hydrated.
- Batch cook, preparing several meals ahead of time.
- If possible, limit store-prepared grab-and-go foods.
- Try to limit your intake of sugars and processed foods.
- Utilize cookbooks for meal-planning ideas.

What to Ask Your Doctor

1. Given my current health status, is there a specific diet you recommend?
2. Are there particular foods you think I should avoid?
3. There's so much information now on carbohydrates being bad for you. What's a reasonable amount of carbohydrates to eat in a day, and what sources do you recommend?

4. Is it okay for me to have dessert? What are some healthier options?

5. Do you recommend I eat organic? Are there certain foods that I should be sure to buy organic?

6. Are there any tests you need to run to make sure I don't have any nutritional deficiencies?

Stay Connected

For many, social connection is a lifeline providing support and comfort in times of intense stress. But over time, caregivers can become isolated, feeling like they are navigating these challenging waters on their own. Sometimes support drops off naturally over time because people are not sure how they can help. Sometimes caregivers stop nurturing their relationships, feeling overwhelmed by their responsibilities. Social isolation can compound grief and lead to increased risk for depression, anxiety, fatigue, and other physical ailments. Just as cancer survivors need a support network to endure the challenges of treatment, caregivers need to stay connected to family, friends, and their community to remain strong and spirited.

Finding time to stay connected and nurture relationships is a critical aspect of a caregiver's self-care. These days, it doesn't have to take a lot of time or even require leaving the house; it is easy to stay connected through email, phone calls, and online video chat services. Seeing someone's face and being able to talk to them in real time can be just as fulfilling, or almost as fulfilling, as meeting in person.

Although long-distance communication is highly valuable, it is still important to make time for in-person connection whenever possible. There is no substitute for being in the physical presence of others. If leaving the house isn't an option, invite people over. If you can get out, do things that you truly enjoy. Perhaps meeting for lunch, coffee, or a walk will provide the sustenance that you need for your body, mind, and inner self. Be discerning about who you spend time with, and seek company that lifts your spirits. After you visit with someone, check in with yourself and see how you are feeling. Was being with that person a supportive, enlivening experience? Remember, this is your precious time and you get to decide how you want to spend it.

What to Do

- Remind yourself that staying connected will help you stay strong for your loved one.

- Plan social connection time on a regular basis—weekly, if possible.

- Use email, phone calls, texting, and video chats for easy ways to connect.

- Consider joining a support group. You can also look online for virtual support groups.

- As much as possible, stay involved in community activities that you enjoy.

- Invite people over. Keep it simple. You don't have to entertain lavishly; just focus on spending time together.

- Accept help when it's offered.

- Consider hiring a caregiver for respite care so you can get out and stay connected.

What to Ask Your Family and Friends

1. Can you possibly come over for a few hours and relieve me so I can get a break?

2. Can you come over for a little while? I may need to keep it on the shorter side, but I'd love to see you.

3. Can we schedule regular check-ins? I don't want to lose touch.

4. I need to go do something fun and would love your company.

5. I would like to attend a support group/class. Can you possibly cover for me so I can attend?

Support Groups

The caregiver's journey can be a lonely one. Although friends and family may kindly offer comfort, there is nothing like the gift of being seen and heard by people who can really identify with what you are going through.

Support groups offer such blessings and much more. For many, the support group becomes a sacred place where they can share thoughts and feelings openly, without judgment, and listen as others impart their experiential knowledge and wisdom. Groups provide a safe forum for questions and concerns. Sometimes you may simply need an understanding ear, and other times you may seek concrete information, direction, and resources or tools for coping with caregiver stress. If you don't wish to share, that's okay. Simply come, listen, and soak in the collective experience.

Groups are a place for you to focus on your own needs and learn about and practice self-care. These discussions can promote self-discovery and empowerment, offering an opportunity to find your voice, learn how to express it, share your wisdom, and feel valued for it. The shared experience of cancer can create strong bonds among group members and allow for special connections and friendships to grow. In going through similar experiences, group members build trust and find comfort and solace.

Support groups are not all created equal. Some groups are for caregivers only, and some are for patients and caregivers to attend together. Some may focus more on education, while others may provide more opportunities for sharing and processing. Each offers its own unique benefits. Contact your cancer care coordinator to find out what groups are offered in your area. You can also contact the American Cancer Society and speak with a representative who can search their database. To find virtual groups, search the Internet for "online support groups for caregivers" and browse the results.

Support groups are worth investigating. Even if you don't typically gravitate toward groups, you may find after attending a couple meetings that the experience resonates with you. Give it a little bit of time and stay open to the process. This may become one of your most valued self-care resources on your caregiving journey.

What to Do

- Talk to your cancer care coordinator to find out about local groups. Ask about the leader's qualifications and how the group is structured and oriented. For example, is the group for caregivers only or for both patients and caregivers?

- If you wish to attend a group, do your best to carve out the time. If needed, ask friends and family to help out by keeping your loved one company while you attend. You can also delegate some tasks to the support network to free up time to attend.

- If transportation is a concern, ask a friend or family member if they can take you. Once you get established, you may be able to ride-share with other members.

- If you prefer to utilize online resources, look online to find out what types of caregiver support groups are available.

What to Ask Your Support Group

1. My loved one struggles with me leaving the house to come to the group. Does anyone else deal with this issue? How do you handle it?

2. I feel guilty taking time for myself. How do you deal with guilt?

3. I feel tired all the time. What can I do to increase my energy?

4. I'm having trouble sleeping. What do other people do for sleep issues?

5. What resources have you found in the community for [your specific issue/question]?

6. What tools do you use to manage stress?

7. Do you have any advice on how to bring up difficult topics of conversation with your loved one?

Be Kind to Yourself

If a dear friend was caretaking and came to you distraught because they felt overwhelmed by all the responsibility and grief-stricken because their loved one was suffering, what would you say? What would you do? How would this make you feel? You would probably feel a lot of compassion, offer your listening ear, and ask how you can help. You would likely think of kind and understanding things to say to make your friend feel seen and heard. You might also suggest they do some things to take care of themselves so they can stay mentally and physically well. You might share that you are concerned for their well-being and help them problem-solve ways to get more help and support.

Now, *you* are the caregiver facing the same responsibilities. How do you speak to yourself? What do you expect of yourself? How well do you take care of yourself?

For some, self-compassion does not come naturally and must be cultivated through conscious practice. Watch how you speak to yourself. Could you be more kind, loving, and accepting? When you get upset or feel impatient with yourself, be forgiving, knowing you are doing your best. If guilt arises, let yourself have those feelings and be understanding and empathetic, just as you would with a friend. Try to speak more positively to yourself to quell your inner critic, recognizing all you do and the efforts you are making to hold everything together. If perfection is your goal, rethink how you can still do a good job without putting such unrealistic expectations on yourself. There may be days when things don't get accomplished exactly how you planned; let that be okay. Remind yourself you are human and you do not have limitless energy.

The more loving caregivers can be toward themselves, the better equipped they will be to continue on their heroic journey.

What to Do

- Make a list of all the things that bring you joy. Pick one item each day and make this your "me" time.

- Bring mindfulness into your everyday life. Mindfulness is achieved by bringing your awareness to the present moment rather than the past or the future. Take a few moments to sit quietly. Thank yourself for everything that you do and are. Intentionally send loving energy and compassion to yourself.

- Ensure that you take breaks.

- Do something fun, such as going to a movie, having a meal out, or getting a nurturing treatment.

- Incorporate social connection into your week.

What to Ask Yourself

1. What makes me feel energized?

2. What brings me feelings of peace and calm?

3. What nice thing can I do for myself today?

4. What's one positive thing I can tell myself?

5. What do I feel grateful for?

6. Who do I enjoy spending time with?

7. What can I eat today that would feel healthy and nurturing?

8. What can I do to incorporate movement today?

9. Would it be helpful if I reached out and connected with someone today?

How Are You Doing?

The Merriam-Webster dictionary definition of *hero* is "a mythical or legendary figure, often of divine descent, endowed with great strength and ability; an illustrious warrior; a person admired for achievements and noble qualities; one who shows great courage."

You could exchange the word *hero* with *caregiver* and the definition would remain the same.

When caregivers are first called into this role, they are embarking on a journey without a road map. Their path leads them to places of beauty and light, as well as darkness and despair. Caregivers learn that they possess strength and courage they never knew they had and can face any adversity one moment at a time. They also recognize that life is so much better and less lonely when they can share their heavy load with those who love and support them. They gain awareness that their bodies are not machines and that their emotions need care and attention. They come to value self-care and recognize the need to be kind to themselves. Caregivers discover that, even in their darkest moments, they are grateful for all the qualities they possess that make it possible for them to endure the challenges they face.

Take a few moments to think about your amazing gifts and express thanks for them. Thank your body, mind, and heart for the job they do for you and your loved one every day. Honor and celebrate the hero that lies in you.

Resources

AgingCare.com
Resources for in-home care, assisted living, and caregiver support.

Cancer.gov
Information on cancer types, screening, diagnosis, staging, treatment types and side effects, clinical trials, and research.

Cancer.net
ASCO-approved information on various types of cancer, coping with cancer, research, and survivorship.

Cancer.org
The American Cancer Society provides a wealth of information on many cancer-related topics, including a breakdown of different types of cancer, treatments, and side effects.

CancerCare.org
Professional oncology counseling, case management, support groups, and workshops.

CancerSupportCommunity.org
Helps caregivers connect with online and local support and offers a cancer support helpline and educational materials.

CaregiverSupportServices.com
Caregiver support, with a focus on wellness resources.

CareZone.com
Tips on organizing health information and medications, with platforms and apps that can provide helpful reminders and other health-care assistance.

Caring.com
Information on estate planning, procuring in-home care, long-term care placement, insurance, and coping with stress and burnout.

CaringBridge.org
Helps those confronting illness stay connected with friends and family and organize support.

Chemocare.com
Information on chemotherapy, related drugs, and managing side effects.

GoodRx.com
Affordable prescriptions through manufacturer prescription savings programs and coupons.

HealthCare.gov
Information on patient protection and the Affordable Care Act.

HospiceCommunityCare.org
Information on hospice care and caregiver resources, including bereavement resources.

LegalTemplates.net
Estate documents, like wills and power of attorney forms.

NCCN.org
The national standard for practice guidelines in oncology, with NCCN guidelines presented in a patient-friendly format.

References

"The AARP Planning Guide for Families and Caregivers." n.d. AARP. Accessed February 29, 2021. AARP.org/caregiving /basics/?intcmp=GLBNAV-SL-CAR-BAS.

"Advanced Cancer." 2015. National Cancer Institute. Accessed January 27, 2021. Cancer.gov/about-cancer/advanced-cancer.

"Anxiety and Cancer." n.d. Chemocare.com. Accessed January 25, 2021. Chemocare.com/chemotherapy/side-effects/anxiety -and-cancer.aspx.

"Cancer and Chemo-based Lack of Appetite and Early Satiety." n.d. Chemocare.com. Accessed January 25, 2021. Chemocare.com/chemotherapy/side-effects/cancer -and-chemobased-lack-of.aspx.

"Cancer Basics." n.d. American Cancer Society. Accessed February 6, 2021. Cancer.org/cancer/cancer-basics.html.

"Care at Home." n.d. AARP. Accessed February 20, 2021. AARP.org/caregiving/home-care/?intcmp=GLBNAV -SL-CAR-CAH.

"Caregiver Burnout: Steps for Coping with Stress." May 14, 2020. AARP. Accessed February 10, 2021. AARP.org/caregiving /life-balance/info-2019/caregiver-stress-burnout .html?intcmp=AE-CAR-CLB-R4-C2.

"Caregiving." n.d. National Institutes of Health. Accessed January 14, 2021. NIA.NIH.gov/health/caregiving.

"Causes and Prevention." 2014. National Cancer Institute. Accessed January 27, 2021. Cancer.gov/about-cancer /causes-prevention.

"Central Neurotoxicity, Memory Loss, and Their Relationship to Chemotherapy." n.d. Chemocare.com. Accessed January 25, 2021. Chemocare.com/chemotherapy/side-effects /central-neurotoxicity-memory-loss.aspx.

"Constipation and Chemotherapy." n.d. Chemocare.com. Accessed January 25, 2021. Chemocare.com/chemotherapy /side-effects/constipation-and-chemotherapy.aspx.

"Coping with Cancer." 2012. Cancer.net. Accessed March 9, 2021. Cancer.net/coping-with-cancer.

"Definition of Hero." n.d. Merriam-Webster. Accessed March 9, 2021. Merriam-Webster.com/dictionary/hero.

"Depression and Chemotherapy." n.d. Chemocare.com. Accessed January 25, 2021. Chemocare.com/chemotherapy/side-effects /depression-and-chemotherapy.aspx.

"Diarrhea and Chemotherapy." n.d. Chemocare.com. Accessed January 25, 2021. Chemocare.com/chemotherapy/side-effects /diarrhea-and-chemotherapy.aspx.

"End of Life Care." n.d. American Cancer Society. Accessed February 6, 2021. Cancer.org/treatment/end-of-life-care.html.

"Fatigue and Cancer Fatigue." n.d. Chemocare.com. Accessed January 25, 2021. Chemocare.com/chemotherapy/side-effects /fatigue-and-cancer.aspx.

"Feelings and Cancer." 2014. National Cancer Institute. February 12, 2014. Accessed January 27, 2021. Cancer.gov/about-cancer /coping/feelings.

"Free Power of Attorney Form." n.d. LegalTemplates. Accessed February 9, 2021. LegalTemplates.net/form/power-of-attorney.

Gregory, Christina, PhD. "The Five Stages of Grief: An Examination of the Kubler-Ross Model." n.d. Psycom. Accessed February 20, 2021. Psycom.net/depression.central.grief.html.

"Guidelines for Patients." n.d. National Comprehensive Cancer Network. Accessed March 1, 2021. NCCN.org/patientresources/patient-resources/guidelines-for-patients.

"Hair Loss and Chemotherapy." n.d. Chemocare.com. Accessed January 25, 2021. Chemocare.com/chemotherapy/side-effects/hair-loss-and-chemotherapy.aspx.

Mustian, Karen M., Lisa K. Sprod, Jennifer Carroll. "Exercise for the Management of Side Effects and Quality of Life Among Cancer Survivors." *Current Sports Medicine Reports* 8, no. 6 (November–December 2009): 325–330. DOI: 10.1249/JSR.0b013e318c22324.

"Nausea, Vomiting, and Chemotherapy." n.d. Chemocare.com. Accessed January 25, 2021. Chemocare.com/chemotherapy/side-effects/nausea-vomiting-chemotherapy.aspx.

"Navigating Cancer Care." 2012. Cancer.net. Accessed March 9, 2021. Cancer.net/navigating-cancer-care.

"Pain and Chemotherapy." n.d. Chemocare.com. Accessed January 25. 2021. Chemocare.com/chemotherapy/side-effects/pain-and-chemotherapy.aspx.

"Personal Finance and Financial Basics." n.d. Fidelity. Accessed February 10, 2021. Fidelity.com/financial-basics/overview.

"Risk Factors for Cancer." 2015. National Cancer Institute. Accessed January 27, 2021. Cancer.gov/about-cancer/causes-prevention/risk.

"Sleep Problems." n.d. Chemocare.com. Accessed January 25, 2021. Chemocare.com/chemotherapy/side-effects /sleep-problems.aspx.

"Symptoms of Cancer." 2015. National Cancer Institute. May 3, 2015. Accessed January 27, 2021. Cancer.gov/about-cancer /diagnosis-staging/symptoms.

"Types of Cancer Treatment." 2017. National Cancer Institute. Accessed January 27, 2021. Cancer.gov/about-cancer /treatment/types.

"Types of Palliative Care." February 2019. Cancer.net. Accessed March 9, 2021. Cancer.net/coping-with-cancer/physical -emotional-and-social-effects-cancer/types-palliative-care.

"Understanding Your Diagnosis." n.d. American Cancer Society. Accessed February 6, 2021. Cancer.org/treatment /understanding-your-diagnosis.html.

Vaughan, Camille P., Patricia S. Goode, Kathryn L. Burgio, and Alayne D. Markland. 2011. "Urinary Incontinence in Older Adults: Urinary Incontinence in Older Adults." *The Mount Sinai Journal of Medicine*, New York 78 (4): 558–570.

"What Causes Cancer?" n.d. American Cancer Society. Accessed February 6, 2021. Cancer.org/cancer/cancer-causes.html.

"What Is Cancer?" 2007. National Cancer Institute. Accessed January 27, 2021. Cancer.gov/about-cancer/understanding /what-is-cancer.

"What is the Financial Treatment Program?" 2020. Family Reach. Accessed February 11, 2021. FamilyReach.org/ftp.

Index

Acknowledgments

I would like to express my deepest gratitude to the extraordinary caregivers who graciously shared their personal stories, bringing life to these pages: Pamela Byers, Valerie Camozzi, Tom Fox, Lori and Michael Haralambidis, Lynn McCloskey, Ilene Pearce, Andrew Rich, Barbara Rich, Alissa Robinow, Denise Wells, Cynthia Wuco, Rafael Yglesias, and Linda Zanko. My sincere thanks to my esteemed oncology colleagues, Dr. Daniel Maloney, David Martin, and Dionne Detraz, for sharing their professional expertise and wisdom. I also wish to give special thanks to my dear friend Barbie Heit for her invaluable contributions and support, and to my editor, Jesse Aylen, for his skill, care, and compassion. And a most heartfelt thank-you to my family and friends, with a special nod to Heidi Pucel and Louis Cheregotis, and to my beloved husband, Gery Hager, for his loving presence and endless support.

About the Author

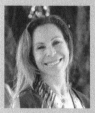 **Victoria Landes, LCSW,** has worked in the medical field for 30 years. Vicki's experience in cancer care dates back to her early career, when she served as a hospice social worker and bereavement counselor. Since then, she has worked in various medical arenas, including hospitals, integrative medical clinics, and outpatient oncology care clinics. More recently, Vicki served as the breast care coordinator for Kaiser Permanente for 12 years, where she accompanied breast cancer survivors and their loved ones through the diagnosis, treatment, and survivorship phases of care. Vicki feels deeply honored to have the opportunity to share the knowledge, wisdom, and insights she has gained from the extraordinary and inspirational people she has met throughout her career.

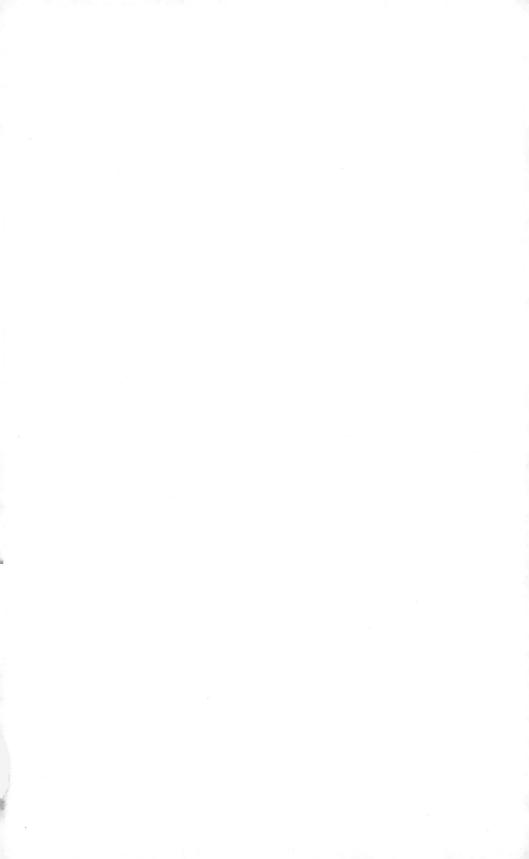

CPSIA information can be obtained
at www.ICGtesting.com
Printed in the USA
JSHW052110070821
17589JS00007B/7